# GREAT MEDICAL DISASTERS

OCT    1989

# GREAT MEDICAL DISASTERS

## DR. RICHARD GORDON

**Author of**
*Doctor in the House*

**DORSET PRESS/New York**

First published in the United States of America in 1983
Copyright ©1983 by Richard Gordon Limited
All rights reserved, Stein and Day, Incorporated

This edition published by Dorset Press,
a division of
Marboro Books Corporation,
by arrangement with
Stein and Day, Incorporated.

1986 Dorset Press.

Library of Congress Cataloging in Publication Data

Gordon, Richard, 1921-
  Great medical disasters.

  Bibliography: p.
  1. Medicine—Anecdotes, facetiae, satire, etc.
1. Title. [DNLM: 1. History of medicine.   2. Mal-
practice—History. W 44 G664g]
R705.G65   1983        610        82-42758

ISBN 0-88029-085-4
(Formerly ISBN 0-8128-2911-5)

Printed in the United States of America
M9 8 7 6

Physicians of all men are most happy; what good success soever they have, the world proclaimeth, and what faults they commit, the earth covereth.

*—Francis Quarles*

Doctors pour drugs of which they know little, to cure diseases of which they know less, into human beings of whom they know nothing.

*—Voltaire*

The medical profession has not a high character; it has an infamous character.

*—Bernard Shaw*

Medicine is a rather philistine sort of profession; it's so often used to acquire rank and status. So many people are attracted to medicine because it will guarantee they will always be respected and important to society.

*—Dr. Jonathan Miller*

The medical is an invidious profession. When one's practice is among the rich one looks like a lackey, when it's among the poor like a thief.

*—Dr. Louis-Ferdinand Céline*

Medicine is an art founded on conjecture and improved by murder.

*—Sir Anthony Carlisle*

> See one physician like a sculler plies
> The patient lingers and by inches dies.
> But two physicians like a pair of oars
> Waft him more swiftly to the Stygian shores.
>
> *—Anon*

He that sinneth before his Maker, let him fall into the hand of the physician.

*—Ecclesiasticus, 38:15.*

Doctors are professional and graduated homicides.

*—Sydney Smith*

Doctors is all swabs.

*—Billy Bones in* Treasure Island

# ACKNOWLEDGMENTS

To the Wellcome Institute for the History of Medicine, the library of the Royal College of Surgeons of England and the London Library.

To the Editor of *Punch*, for kind permission to reproduce the verse in *Doctor Death*.

# CONTENTS

## PART TEN: Final Diagnosis

# A DISASTROUS PRACTICE

Thousands of books have been published on the triumphs of medicine.

This is the other one.

Medicine has its Tampa Bay Bridge, Titanic, Great Fire of London, and San Francisco Earthquake.

Even its equivalents of pussycats up trees, burst watermains and thunderstorms are major disasters if they happen to *you*.

Mankind suffered cruelly for centuries from lack of medical knowledge. The brilliant scientific discoveries of this century eradicated the evil so efficiently it now suffers as painfully from too much.

Doctors can be fired by ideals—as fanatically as the Spanish Inquisition. They can follow more false trails than Inspector Clouseau. They can become so fond of dead doctrines, they resemble a procession of ostriches with their heads in the sand.

The medical art is revealed by its disasters, as the military one is by its defeats.

This catalogue of disasters will make you feel great to be alive.

# Part One

# DISASTROUS DOCTORS

# 1

## TRIPLE KNOCK-OUT

### Disastrous Surgical Enthusiasm

Robert Liston was the fastest knife in the West End. He could amputate a leg in 2½ minutes.

He lived during the 1840s at No. 5 Clifford Street, off Bond Street in Mayfair. His three-story house with tall downstairs windows, elegantly spiralling oak staircase and boot-scraper, now faces the club that invented Buck's fizz.

Liston was an incorrigible bustler, even for a surgeon. He eschewed carriages, visited his patients on horseback, and loved hunting. His reputation for speedy wizardry so choked his waiting room, the butler had to circulate a reviving decanter of madeira and biscuits. When anesthesia was unknown—you had the choice of fuddling with opium or rum, or biting on a cloth-wrapped peg—surgery was a matter of more haste, less pain.

He was six foot two, and operated in a bottle-green coat with Wellington boots. He sprung across the bloodstained boards upon his swooning, sweating, strapped-down patient like a duelist, calling, "Time me, gentlemen, time me!" to students craning with pocket watches from the iron-railinged galleries. Everyone swore that the first flash of his knife was followed so swiftly by the rasp of saw on bone that sight and sound seemed simultaneous. To free both hands, he would clasp the bloody knife between his teeth.

Liston invented see-through isinglass adhesive tape, the "bulldog" artery forceps, and a leg splint still used during World War II. The son of a Scots minister, he graduated from Edinburgh, became first "The Great Northern Anatomist" of *Blackwood's Magazine,* was rumored enthusiastically to "resurrect" his own corpses.

An abrupt, abrasive, argumentative man, unfailingly charitable to the poor and tender to the sick, impossibly vain, he was vilely unpopular among his fellow surgeons at the Edinburgh Royal Infirmary. He relished operating successfully in the reeking tenements of the Grassmarket and Lawnmarket on patients they had discharged as hopelessly incurable. They conspired to bar him from the wards, banishing him South where he became professor of surgery at University College Hospital in London and made a fortune.

It was Robert Liston who performed, on December 21, 1846, the first operation under anesthesia in Europe. Only comment: "This Yankee dodge beats mesmerism hollow." The leg hit the sawdust in the bucket after 2½ minutes, but his talent for surgical velocity was already outdated.

### Liston's fourth most famous case

Removal in four minutes of a 45-pound scrotal tumor, whose owner had to carry it around in a wheelbarrow.

### Liston's third most famous case

Argument with his intern. Was the red, pulsating tumor in a small boy's neck a straightforward abscess of the skin? Or a dangerous aneurism of the carotid artery? "Pooh!" Liston exclaimed impatiently. "Whoever heard of an aneurism in a boy so young?" Flashing a knife from his waistcoat pocket, he lanced it. Intern's note: "Out leaped arterial blood, and the boy fell." The patient died but the artery lives, in the University College Hospital pathology museum, specimen No. 1256.

### Liston's second most famous case

Amputated the leg in 2½ minutes, but in his enthusiasm the patient's testicles as well.

### Liston's most famous case

Amputated the leg *under* 2½ minutes (the patient died afterward in the ward from hospital gangrene, they usually did in those pre-Listerian days). He amputated in addition, the fingers of his young assistant (who died afterward in the ward from hospital gangrene, they usually did in those pre-Listerian days). He also slashed through the coattails of a distinguished surgical spectator, who was so terrified that the knife had pierced his vitals he dropped dead from fright.

That was the only operation in history with a 300 percent mortality.

# 2

# THE EMPEROR'S SORE THROAT
## Sir Morell Mackenzie and the Kaiser

At Queen Victoria's Jubilee in 1887, the world looked as beautiful for Germany as fifty-three years later. Denmark had been crushed, Austria pulverized, and France flattened.

*Reichskanzler* Bismarck ran an unflinchingly efficient empire bossed by Prussia. The crown princess was Victoria's eldest child, "Viki." Her 30-year-old son, William—his left arm was paralyzed from an undiagnosed birth injury—was Victoria's favorite grandchild. To the queen of England, foreign affairs were family affairs, conducted with letters full of state secrets to eight of her nine children married into European courts.

The German Emperor William I had turned 90. Viki's husband, Frederick, compassionate, democratic, earnest, war-hating, intended to thwart Bismarck and rule the 39 German states linked in peaceful, liberal brotherhood. Princess Viki thought anyone mad who was blind to the overpowering advantages of the British Constitution. She was *die Engländerin,* distrusted and hated. William of the upswept mustaches was Prussian from the spike of his helmet to the click of his heels and fitted comfortably into Bismarck's tunic pocket.

Among these royalties was dropped a pigheaded, humorless, self-satisfied, pushful, touchy middle-aged Scot, who beheld the world through a shilling-sized throat mirror.

That January, stolid, bearded 55-year-old Crown Prince Frederick grew hoarse. It was ascribed to a nasty cold when his coachman became lost in the dark among the mountains, and the prince had no overcoat. The aromatic inhalations, the tangy gargles, were useless. His physician, Dr. Wegner, Deputy Medical-Director of the German army, called in Professor Gerhardt, the throat man from Berlin.

The professor sprayed cocaine and observed through his mirror a pink nodule on the left vocal chord. He tried pulling it off with a wire snare. No good. He thrust down a knife. No good, either. He sent for the electric cautery and sizzled. The lump got bigger. The professor attacked with the cautery every day for a fortnight. Frederick's motto was *Lerne zu leiden ohne zu klagen*— we must learn to suffer without complaint.

The wound refused to heal. The professor thought vaguely of cancer. But the vocal chords moved normally, which every doctor at the time knew excluded malignancy. Every doctor at the time was disastrously wrong. He prescribed a fortnight at a spa.

The hoarseness grew worse. Gerhardt decided to split open the Adam's apple and look. He called in Professor von Bergmann to do the cutting (physicians then utilizing surgeons as householders do plumbers). The operation was fixed among the doctors for 7 A.M. on Saturday, May 21. With a stealth appropriate to high crimes and misdemeanors, operating table and nurses were brought from the Charité Hospital in Berlin to the Neue Palais at Potsdam, which had no bathrooms.

Bismarck discovered with fury they were about to chloroform the Heir-Apparent without telling himself, the old emperor, or even the patient. He instantly dispatched reinforcements, Dr. Schrader, Professor Tobold, Dr. Hahn and Dr. von Lauer, who could pull rank as Dr. Wegner's commander in the army. Uneasy lies the head that wears a crown, on a pillow with a circus of doctors around it.

Late that night, Queen Victoria's doctor James Reid, an Aberdonian who resembled a bewhiskered hard-boiled egg, appeared unexpectedly in Dr. Morell Mackenzie's bric-a-brac stuffed consulting room at No. 19, Harley Street, London.

The queen had passed a frightful day. Two frantic telegrams, a distracted letter from Viki, revealed the alarming intention of removing a suspicious, perhaps cancerous, growth in the throat of *unser Fritz*. Viki implored instant dispatch of the celebrated Dr. Mackenzie. "We cannot bear to think of poor darling Viki's anguish and sorrow," cried the queen. (She was far more emotional, more vivacious than the statue of her memory. Her evergreen rod, "We are not amused" swished an equerry telling a spicy story over dinner at Windsor—but maybe he had been loyally following her Majesty's habit of lacing her claret with Scotch.)

The German doctors had already startled Mackenzie that afternoon with a telegram to join the team. Perhaps they wanted to dilute responsibility. Perhaps they recognized he knew more about the throat than they did. To travel in the purple of the queen's authority he found electrifying.

Mackenzie was sharp-nosed, thin-lipped, hollow-cheeked, neatly sidewhiskered, in wing collar and frock coat. He smelt of stramonium, taken in cigarettes for his asthma. His practice was so busy, urgent patients needed to tip his butler for priority. In 1887, you lost your tonsils sitting conscious in a high-backed chair, the operator wandering off to puff a throat with powder, to prescribe a gargle or two, before reappearing to mop up the blood.

Mackenzie's dinner table attracted Henry Irving, Beerbohm Tree, Ellen Terry, Pinero, and James McNeill Whistler (Whistler's mother's other son was a London throat doctor). His profession despised him as an adventurer. The Royal College of Surgeons regarded his Throat Hospital—still flourishing at Golden Square in Soho—as the Bank of England a pawnbroker's.

Arrived at Potsdam, Mackenzie plunged his own forceps down the patient's throat. The fragments went to Professor Virchow, the world-famous pathologist who discovered leukemia, abominated Bismark, and relaid the Berlin drains. Virchow looked down his microscope and pronounced no cancer. Mackenzie cancelled the operation and went home.

His patient followed in June, for three months' Jubilee celebrations. Mackenzie continued to pick away at his larynx with forceps, as a bird at a nut. On September 7, Queen Victoria summoned Mackenzie to Balmoral and knighted him in the drawing room after lunch.

The crown prince wintered among the flowers and palms of

San Remo on the Italian Riviera. On November 5, Mackenzie had a telegraphed summons to the Villa Zirio. The lump had grown frighteningly, spreading to the opposite vocal chord. "Is it cancer?" asked the crown prince, in his whisper. Mackenzie answered, "I am sorry to say, sir, it looks very much like it." He had, in May, clumsily plucked a speck of normal tissue for Professor Virchow. Frederick gave a sad smile. "Under the circumstances I really must apologize for feeling so well."

The relations of doctors and the press were simple in the 1880s. You told the scoundrels nothing. The outraged German papers had blazed all summer at the crown princess, for thrusting an English doctor against a future German emperor's sickbed. San Remo was full of reporters, ambushing Mackenzie and training telescopes on the villa. The thunder of *The Times* rolled across the Channel.

The doctors started quarrelling with Mackenzie more openly than with each other. They became a round dozen with the arrival of Professor von Schrötter from Vienna, Dr. Krause from Berlin, and Dr. Mark Hovell from Golden Square. Unlucky thirteen was Dr. Moritz Schmidt, hurried from Frankfurt by Prince William, who had decided to take charge of the case himself.

William paraded the doctors. How long had his father to live? Eighteen months, said Mackenzie. How long had the cancer been there? Dr. Krause volunteered, six months. "I thought Mackenzie would die of shame!" exclaimed the future Kaiser. "But his face, which I was watching narrowly, showed no trace of emotion."

His mother disagreed. "I cannot enough repeat how wise and kind, how delicate and considerate and judicious Sir Morell Mackenzie is," she wrote to Queen Victoria. Her husband faced his doctors' alternatives. He could have his whole larynx excised immediately, which was more likely to be an assassination attempt than an operation. Or he could have a simple tracheostomy hole to breathe through, whenever necessary in the indefinite future. He chose the second. He was the calmest man in the room.

The press would be left in a mist, from which the hard facts could emerge gradually. The public grew as petulant as children kept from adults' secrets. William made the doctors sign a confidential bulletin admitting the truth, which in a couple of days leaked into the Berlin papers. In Berlin coffeehouses they recalled the Salic Law, forbidding succession to the throne through the female line—Queen Victoria would otherwise have been also Queen of Hanover. It was muttered that the Hohenzollern family had a similar rule excluding the weak and sickly. Bismark already had the doddery emperor authorize young William's signing state papers in his father's stead, and planned to proclaim him regent on his grandfather's death.

The gentle patient gently got worse. At 3 P.M. on January 9, 1888, the operation plotted the previous May was performed in the Villa Zirio's drawing room by a young Dr. Bramann, who was experienced in tracheostomies for children choking with diphtheria. Mackenzie issued a statement to the *Lancet* saying the disease was not cancer. Well, probably not. His daughter Ethel came from London and inflamed the German newspapers by playing tennis with Viki's daughter, and particularly as they had discovered Mackenzie to be really a Polish Jew called Moritz Marcovicz.

The patient's strength declined. The doctors' increased. Professors Kaussmaul and Waldeyer made sixteen. On March 9, the old Emperor William I died. The voiceless new one, Frederick III, took train through the Alpine snowstorms to Berlin. Everyone said that Bismark arranged it, hoping the journey would kill him.

April 12 was a terrible afternoon. The tracheostomy hole Frederick breathed through always needed a curved metal tube inside. Mackenzie was inserting a better design, and thought it tactful to invite Professor von Bergmann to the Neue Palais from Berlin. The galloping messenger traced him to a hotel. He was drunk. (He had pinned the aristocratic "von" to his name. He was no Prussian, but a Slav from Riga, where they were notorious martyrs to the bottle.) He insisted on operating himself. He poked the tube into the neck muscles. The patient went blue. He followed it with his forefinger. The emperor nearly died. The doctors scurrilously blamed each other, in private and the press. Queen Victoria arrived, and scolded Prince William for unfilial behavior. Professor Leyden, Professor Senator, Dr. Landgret, and Professor Bardeleben of the Charité brought the medical squad to twenty. The emperor started coughing up his own windpipe. After 93 days' reign, he died of bronchopneumonia.

The new Kaiser William II posted armed guards at all entrances and patrols of hussars in the grounds, forebade anyone to leave or send a telegram on pain of arrest, ransacked his father's private papers. Viki begged in tears that her husband be spared the defilement of a postmortem. William insisted. They sewed him up just in time for the lying-in-state. Over-manned to the last, he was anatomized by ten doctors.

Mackenzie left Germany with a £12,000 fee, the hate of the people, and the spite of the press. The kaiser and Bismarck accused him of deliberately concealing the diagnosis, so that Frederick might escape being declared incapable of reigning. Perhaps they were right. Frederick chose at San Remo the unimpending risk, which promised brief rule to establish a government and reward politically slighted friends (Mackenzie got the Hohenzollern Cross and Star).

Bismarck's son, the foreign minister, asserted the emperor would have lived for years without the misfortune of meeting Mackenzie. The German doctors castigated Mackenzie for stopping the May operation, which they wishfully insisted would have cured the disease. The German people more earthily accused him of ensuring the fatter empress's pension for *die Engländerin*, who once possessed of her dowry was going to marry her chamberlain Count Seckendorff. Everyone knew it for a fact.

Mackenzie retaliated. He sued *The Times* and the *St. James's Gazette* for libel. In *The Fatal Illness of Frederick the Noble* he justified himself as Oliver Twist in a medical Fagin's kitchen. The book appeared in the lurid autumn of Jack the Ripper.

The public refused his dose of vitriol. Reviewers and editors were revolted by a quarrel over a corpse. The Royal College of Surgeons disparaged him for violating the secrets of the sick room—as Lord Moran 78 years later, after Churchill's deathbed. The Royal College of Physicians, whom Mackenzie had called "an academy of decorous mediocrity," paid off old scores and made him resign. He stood amazed amid the shattered eggshell of his self-righteousness. He passed Whistler's presentation copy of *The Gentle Art of Making Enemies* to his assistant: "I do not seem to have any need to study it." Two years later he was dead, aged fifty-four.

Mackenzie's expedition was a disaster, clinically, professionally, and politically. The doctors applied to a disease of which they knew little, treatment of which they should have been ashamed. It was an unusual case. The cancer supervened on another condition.

In this year of Frederick's death, *Drame Impérial* was published by Jean de Bonnefon, who had covered San Marino for the Paris newspaper *Gaulois*. He asserted that the crown prince had syphilis. The prince had caught it from a delicious *señorita* Dolores Cada. She was part of the celebrations at the opening of the Suez Canal in 1869. The Khedive's physician treated him sketchily, Frederick returned to the tedium of being a dutiful husband. *Mais le germe n'était pas mort, il dormait.* Not dead, but sleepeth. When Mackenzie told Viki the correct diagnosis, she slapped his face.

The doctors at San Remo gave antisyphilitic treatment with potassium iodide, as gleefully discovered by the French papers. Mackenzie explained forcefully it was prescribed only *to exclude* —and since there was no cure, clearly there was no syphilis. Professor von Schrötter scoffed at an *altes Weibergeschwätz*, old wives' tale. Frederick was certainly syphilitic. A throat surgeon I knew as an intern learned the secret from Mackenzie's most intimate friend. Mackenzie's reputation was attacked for what he did not say—that the emperor had cancer, while he suffered from what he could not—that the emperor had syphilis.

No Victorian doctor could have saved the Emperor. Had God not pressed His cancerous thumbprint for another ten years, perhaps democracy would have rooted in Germany, the mighty German army and magnificent British fleet peacefully policed the world, Kaiser William grown to wiser ways. Instead, Queen Victoria died in the Kaiser's arms, and three-quarter million of her countrymen in his defiance.

# 3

## KINKY KINKS

### *Corset Disaster*

> Your nuciform sac is full of decaying matter—undigested food and
> waste products—rank ptomaines. Now you take my advice, Rid-
> geon. Let me cut it out for you. You'll be another man afterwards.

Mr. Cutler Walpole on November 20, 1906, on the stage of the
Court Theater, London. The play was Shaw's *Doctor's Dilemma*.

Across the Thames, Sir William Arbuthnot Lane, Bt., starred
in the theater of Guy's Hospital.

Many are obsessed with their bowels. Sir William was
obsessed with the bowels of the whole world. The colon—the last
lap of the guts—he saw coiled in the abdomen like a snake in the
grass. A static, solid, seething sac of putrifying provisions, its
poisons absorbed by the bloodstream to ruin physical and psycho-
logical health. Constipation! Chronic intestinal stasis! Auto-
intoxication! he diagnosed frenzedly. He described an everyday
case.

> The sensation imparted to the hand of the observer by that of the
> toxic patient is unmistakable. It is cold and clammy, and moist on
> its palmar surface. The ears are also bluish and feel cold, as also
> does the nose. . . . The loss of fat in the face and neck produces an
> appearance of age, distress, and disappointment which is most

pathetic, particularly in the young subject. . . . The individual is also unable to lead an active physical life because of poor muscular development.

He also had "a nasty graveyard odour."

Sir William Lane reads much like Dr. William Acton (see Chapter 40, Disastrous Habits). If the patients masturbated as well, God knows what they looked like.

The colon was perpetually loaded, how could he rid it of feces? He tried a pint of cream a day, and so much liquid paraffin that a match applied to the fundament would have illuminated the drawing room. He had men wear body-belts, ladies change their corsets. "The English corset is disastrous. . . . The straight-busked French corset is much less harmful."

Then he discovered Lane's kink, and surgically shortcircuited it. Fair enough. Had you taken your symptoms to the man next door in Cavendish Square, he would as eagerly have anchored your floating kidneys, buoyed up your sinking stomach, or divided your invisible adhesions. Doctors are slaves to fashion as much as dress designers.

In the 1900s, Lane met Elie Metchnikoff, Russian Nobel Prize winner. Metchnikoff had written a book proving the entire one-and-a-half yards of colon a useless, vestigial structure, like the appendix. It was the meeting of pope and crusader. Lane afterward removed his patients' colons as nonchalantly as he shook their clammy hands. A boy misdirected from a throat surgeon had his colon removed instead of his tonsils. A man who tried cutting his throat nearly had his wife's colon removed, to better her temper and reduce domestic suicidal pressure.

Sir William had his critics. "Encouraged by us doctors," declared another medical knight just before World War I, "hundreds and thousands of human beings have grafted into themselves the idea that they were born into the world for the main purpose of getting a daily evacuation of their bowels, for should they fail in this they will be poisoned by the absorption of the noxious products that are, they suppose, forming in this their kitchen garden.

The garden grew Sir William £10,000 a year.

Lane died during World War II aged 86, outliving his operation by thirty years. He was not Cutler Walpole of the fictional nuci-form sac. Shaw confessed his original "a laryngeal specialist who extirpated uvulas." Which is equally effective treatment for con-stipation, a meaningless term depending wholly on personal standards, like insomnia and pornography.

# 4

## THE TENDER TRAP

### Delicate Disaster

The solution for male doctors who do rough pelvic exams on women might begin in medical schools, where each male student would be placed in stirrups and a strange female M.D. would come and "squeeze his balls and leave without saying a word." That's the advice of Dr. Joan Magee, a gynecologist, writing in the *Annals of Internal Medicine*.

—*Chatelaine Magazine*

# 5

## SURGICAL SOUVENIRS

### *Litigious Litter*

These operative oversights were reported to a doctors' legal insurance society in London for a period of 18 years.

| | Swabs Left Inside | All Articles (instruments, needles, etc.) Left Inside |
|---|---|---|
| 1962 | 38 | 41 |
| 1963 | 27 | 45 |
| 1964 | 37 | 68 |
| 1965 | 32 | 54 |
| 1966 | 31 | 52 |
| 1967 | 30 | 41 |
| 1968 | 26 | 39 |
| 1969 | 25 | 46 |
| 1970 | 21 | 28 |
| 1971 | 33 | 56 |
| 1972 | 31 | 60 |
| 1973 | 25 | 30 |
| 1974 | 20 | 35 |
| 1975 | 25 | 46 |

| | Swabs Left Inside | All Articles (instruments, needles, etc.) Left Inside |
|---|---|---|
| 1976 | 26 | 45 |
| 1977 | 21 | 90 |
| 1978 | 18 | 60 |
| 1979 | 16 | 110 |
| Totals | 482 | 946 |

Surgeons are becoming no less forgetful.

More gruesomely, a large forceps used for holding swabs (acting like scissors with locking handles, measuring nine-and-a-half inches by three) was discovered in the ashes of a woman aged 76 a week after an operation on her kidney. The operation wound itself was much smaller, only five inches long and three-and-a-half inches deep. It could never have concealed the forceps. No instruments were missing in the operating theaters or the sterile supply store. No one ever knew how it accompanied her to the furnace.

Such examples of the almost mystical misplacement of matter are disturbing. But doctor's lives were never serene . . .

# Part Two

# MALPRACTICE MADNESS

# 6

# THE KING IS DEAD

## *Not Without Help*

On the Sunday evening of February 1, 1685, Protestant King Charles II of England, aged 53, sat fondling the Duchesses of Portsmouth, Cleveland, and Mazarin—three of his thirteen mistresses—while a score of his courtiers crouched over a heap of two thousand golden guineas playing basset, a simple game depending on the turn of a card, and a French boy sang love songs.

At eight o'clock the next morning, just out of bed to be shaved, the king uttered a cry and had fits. Dr. Edmund King, a guest at Whitehall Palace, applied emergency treatment by letting sixteen ounces of blood from a vein in the left arm, while messengers were sent galloping for the royal physicians.

The fashionable doctor was becoming the man of fashion—buckskin breeches and silver-buckled shoes, velvet coat and full-bottomed wig, tricorn hat and beaver muff in winter. His essential equipment was a gold-headed cane, its perforated head crammed with aromatic herbs to ward off infection, or at least the stink. The king paid his doctors £100 a year, and they charged half-a-guinea for coffeehouse consultations. Bleeding a lady in bed cost ten shillings, a man half-a-crown, and you could get a postmortem for three-and-fourpence.

Everyday illness meant plague, typhus, or smallpox. Surgery was setting limbs and cutting for gall and kidney stone. The doctors of Europe were restive for new ideas. Harvey had changed the heart from the seat of emotion to a pump (Dr. Jonathan Miller says because pumps were proliferating with the thriving of mining). The Dutch had anatomized and microscoped. At Oxford, they were sniffing out the vital function of oxygen. Health and disease were losing their mystique and becoming as worldly as profit and loss in a City of London counting-house.

Was the body a machine, its teeth scissors, chest bellows, stomach grinding millstones? Or a vat of fermenting juices, to be blended skillfully by the doctors as the brewer his beer? These new philosophies were shot through with immutable superstition.

## TREATMENT FIT FOR A KING

### Monday

Their leader Sir Charles Scarburgh said the six physicians "Flocked quickly to the King's assistance; and after they had held a consultation together, they strenuously endeavoured to afford timely succour to His Majesty in his dangerous state."

Immediately, they applied to his shoulders three cupping-glasses like wineglasses, flamed to expel the air and raise mounds of skin. This treatment was performed in the stone age with animals' horns. Cupping was instantly followed by scarification, for eight ounces of blood.

"Within a few moments of this," recounted Sir Charles, "so as to free his stomach of all impurities, and by the same action to rid his whole nervous system of anything harmful to it, we administered an Emetic." This was antimony in the equivalent of curacoa, but the king jibbed. They gave him vitriol in peony water, a couple of purgative pills, and the clyster.

It was the golden age of the clyster, delivered through the nozzle of a metal syringe, as used for spraying roses. Application and result was such a beautiful demonstration of Descartes' *l'homme-machine*.

"Wind doth now and then torment me about the fundament extremely," complained Pepys, whose wife ministered him one of strong ale, four ounces of sugar, and two ounces of butter. ("Two stools in the night—pissed well.")

The king's was less robustly tasty—mallow leaves, violets, beet, chamomile flowers, fennel seeds, linseed, cinnamon, cardomom, saffron, cochineal, and aloes. It was repeated after two hours, accompanied orally with syrup of blackthorn, more antimony, and some rock salt.

The physicians were impatient. They dropped another charge of purgatives, shaved his hair, and stuck blistering plasters all over his head. The king had more fits. They sent for the red-hot cautery.

Before its arrival, the king luckily regained consciousness. The doctors were ecstatic. How brilliantly their treatment worked! The patient must enjoy more of it.

To relieve the pressure of humors, they purged as a matter of course and excited sneezing with white hellebore root up the nostrils. They gave powdered cowslip flowers to strengthen the brain, then more purgatives to keep the bowels going during the night. The blistering plasters of cantharidin—"Spanish fly," the ageless aphrodisiac—irritated the urinary passages when absorbed through the skin and then excreted. The doctors treated this scalding urine with a soothing decoction of barley, licorice, and sweet almond kernels. The king's supper was thin broth and ale without hops. They plastered the soles of his feet with tar and pigeon-dung, gave him another enema, and said good-night.

### Tuesday

The patient was *much* better! "The blessing of God being approved by the application of proper and seasonable remedies," Sir Charles congratulated the Almighty and himself. They told the king to go on taking the potions.

The doctors were now twelve. This treatment of royalty by committee—persisting disastrously for Frederick of Prussia two hundred years later as we saw in Chapter 2—is ruthlessly rich in bright suggestions. At noon, they opened both jugulars for ten ounces of blood. They gave a gargle of elm in syrup of mallow for his sore throat. To prevent more fits, they prescribed a julep of black cherry, peony, lavender, crushed pearls, and white sugar candy, which sounds lovely.

## Wednesday

The doctors' sunny confidence brought milder draughts of senna pods infused in spring water, given with white wine and nutmeg. At five that afternoon, they issued their first bulletin from the Whitehall Council Chamber for the morrow's *London Gazette*, ending, "that they conceive His Majesty to be in a condition of safety, and that he will in a few days to be freed from his distemper."

## Thursday

When the bulletin appeared, the King was nearly dead. He suddenly had more fits. During the night they gave him a spiritous draft made from the skull of a man who met violent death, the clinical equivalent of extreme unction.

The king's ministers grew anxious and angry. What was His Majesty suffering *from*? The doctors had no idea.

They consulted urgently. Intermittent fever! There was a lot of it about in London that time of year. And they could cure it! Send for the Peruvian bark, quick!

This was chincona bark, full of quinine. It was picturesquely named after the Countess of Chinchon, wife to the Spanish viceroy of Peru, well known to be miraculously cured of malaria by it (in fact, she died of something else in Cartagena, still on her way to Peru). "Jesuits bark" was being dispensed by the Society of Jesus in Lima in the 1630s, and caused Oliver Cromwell severe misgivings to ingest.

They gave it every three hours in milk, interspersed with more human skull.

Neither worked.

## Friday

The king was worse. That night, they had to use Raleigh's Stronger Antidote and Goa Stone. He apologized for being an unconscionable time dying and asked them not to let poor Nelly starve. Toward dawn, they gave the Oriental Bezoar Stone, a rare concretion from the stomach of an East Indian goat. The king grew breathless. He was bled. At eight-thirty in the morning his speech faltered and failed. At ten he was comatose. At noon he died (as a Roman Catholic).

### Saturday

The king was rumored to have been poisoned, but most kings earn that rumor at their dying. A postmortem was held. The brain was engorged with blood, there was old pleurisy of the right lung, the heart was enlarged. Nothing else was wrong. The illness seemed hardly worth all the fuss.

Charles II probably died from high blood pressure, after kidney failure caused by his gout. The treatment neither delayed nor hastened his death, only made it more painful and wretched. His physicians were doing their best, according to their lights. Who dare claim our medical lights today always shine truer than Will o'the Wisp?

# 7

## THE DECLINE AND FALL
## OF EDWARD GIBBON

### *Inexpressible Embarrassment*

Edward Gibbon was fat and foppish. His literary opponents ridiculed both the affliction and the affectation. He also suffered from gout.

He got the idea for *The Decline and Fall of the Roman Empire* in the Capitol ruins at Rome on October 15, 1765, and finished it toward midnight in a summerhouse at Lausanne on June 27, 1787. On November 11, 1793, he wrote from St. James's in London to his friend and editor Lord Sheffield in Sussex:

> I must at length withdraw the veil before my state of health though the naked truth may alarm you more than a fit of the gout. Have you never observed through my *inexpressibles* a large prominency which, as it was not at all painful and very little troublesome I had strangely neglected for many years? But since my departure from Sheffield Place it has increased (most stupendously) is increasing and ought to be diminished. Yesterday I sent for Farquhar who is allowed to be a very skillful surgeon. After viewing and palpating he desired to call in assistance and has examined it again today with Mr. Cline, a surgeon, as he says, of the first eminence. They both pronounce it a hydrocele [a collection of water] which must be let out by the operation of tapping, but from its magnitude and long neglect they think it a most extraordinary

case and wish to have another surgeon, Dr. Baille, present. If the business should go off smoothly I shall be delivered from my burden (it is almost as big as a small child) and walk about in four or five days with a truss. But the medical gentlemen, who never speak quite plain, insinuate to me the possibility of an inflammation, of fever, etc.

It was a disastrous decision.

Hydrocele is a benign and common scrotal condition. The operation performed a few days later produced four quarts of clear fluid, the burden reduced by half. A cruel relief. A fortnight later the lump grew as big as ever, the draining repeated. The fluid again returned, the insinuated inflammation gripped, the operation site was covered with ulcers.

By January 9, 1794, Gibbon ran a high fever. Four days later, the surgeons made a third incision and took six quarts. Next morning he seemed better, the next he suffered sickness and abdominal pain, treated with warm cloths and opium. He rose after a wretched night at eight-thirty, returned to bed for Mr. Farquhar at eleven. The surgeon found his patient collapsed, shook his head, and left. Edward Gibbon took some brandy at noon and three-quarters of an hour later was dead.

He was 56. Had he let well enough alone, he might have lived to the Battle of Waterloo. He could have emulated the treatment of Mr. Robert Liston's patient with the wheelbarrow. He suffered the slowly growing hydrocele for 32 years, since first consulting the surgeon Mr. Hawkins. Had he submitted to eighteenth-century surgery then, much of the world would never have known the grandeur that was Rome, and Gibbon would be remembered as a captain on the rolls of the Hampshire militia.

# 8

## THE SACK-'EM-UP MEN
### Disaster for Scottish Anatomy

"Heal the sick, cleanse the lepers, raise the dead, cast out devils," Jesus sent forth His disciples, knowing of course the forthcoming split of medicine into therapeutics, epidemiology, resuscitation, and psychiatry.

The early Christians obeyed with evangelical zeal. They claimed exclusive world rights in healing, prescribing prayer, and fasting. The human body was sacred, never to be violated by dissection (the Moslems agreed). Religion thus immobilized medicine for fifteen centuries.

A doctor who has never run his fingers through a body is an astronomer without a telescope. Galen in the second century did his best with Barbary apes. The Renaissance anatomist Andreas Versalius founded his career on luckily discovering, outside the walls of Louvain, a criminal's skeleton hanging in chains, complete with ligaments. When Henry VIII decreed in 1540 that surgeons were a cut above barbers, he awarded them two executed criminals a year for dissection.

From gallows and gibbet came medicine's greatest benefactors. Anatomy schools flourished with the hangman in the eighteenth century. Windmill Street in Soho had Scotsman William Hunter's famous Theatre of Anatomy, continuing the tradition two centuries later with London's first strip show. In 1717, Edinburgh appointed its first professor of anatomy, age 22. There was sometimes a wee fret over students posing as mourners and snatching the body. One newly executed woman revived during a fight over hers, and lived on for years as "Half-hangit Maggie."

The official Edinburgh University anatomists suffered competition from able extramural teachers with a robust, showbiz approach, lecturing in a rivalry that infected their devoted students. All needed to keep "the table" adequately furnished. Six taught in Surgeons' Square, by the Infirmary in High School Yards, with its adjoining plot for burying unclaimed bodies. This was to the students an academic convenience as prized as the Bodleian at Oxford.

Snatching a body is easier than catching a salmon:

1. Wait till dark.
2. Post a couple of lookouts against rival resurrectionists and excitable relatives.
3. Dig a hole in the loose earth *at the head* of the grave. Use a flat, daggerlike spade of *wood,* to avoid noise with the stones. Spread canvas sheet for soil, keeping grass uncontaminated.
4. Apply two hooks to coffin lid, pull with rope, splinter lid (pack hole with sacks to muffle cracking noise).
5. Take body *by both ears,* extract.
6. Replace shroud. (That would be stealing. A body belongs to nobody.)
7. Sack up body.
8. Tidy up, remove tools from site, decamp.

It should take an hour.

The most popular anatomist in Edinburgh was Dr. Robert Knox, his rooms a three-story balconied and porticoed house at No. 10 Surgeons' Square, jammed between Surgeons' Hall and the Royal Medical Society. In the winter of 1828 he was teaching 504 pupils, three-quarters of the whole medical school. He was 37, claimed descent from John ("Monstrous Regiment of Women") Knox, had German blood, once treated the wounded at Waterloo, was as much part of the Edinburgh scene as Arthur's Seat.

He was dome-headed and sidewhiskered, sharp-nosed with a

jutting lower lip, chin lost in high collar, festooned with golden watch-chains and seals, a diamond cravat-ring, little round glasses, one-eyed like Mr. Squeers. He was contentious, caustic, cynical, vain, evasive, and spiteful. He lectured his students with relish about Robert Liston mistaking a neck aneurism for an abscess, killing a patient in the next door Infirmary—odd, because they were telling the same story six years later set in London, with the fragment in a jar to prove it (see Chapter 1, Triple Knock-Out). Perhaps Liston made a habit of it.

Knox was an enthusiastic raconteur, a gripping lecturer. He needed to repeat each discourse thrice a day to a crammed lectureroom of applauding students. He loved anatomy as Romeo did Juliet. The fee for the course was £3.5s, extra for "subjects" (guaranteed fresh). For his own demonstrations and his pupils' dissections, Knox had a logistical problem. He was paying £800 a year to sportive students and Edinburgh's lurking resurrectionists.

On the night of November 29, 1827, two new suppliers brought Dr. Knox an old man in a sack and got £7.10s. They had intended taking him to the university's Professor Monro, which would have saved Dr. Knox much later trouble, the couple being Burke and Hare.

The corpse was an army pensioner who had died in Hare's boardinghouse at Tanner's Close in slummy West Port beyond Grassmarket, beneath the castle. He had owed the landlord £4, and lodger Burke agreed the loss could be justifiably cleared by turning the debtor into a "shot for the doctor." They cracked open the coffin, popped the corpse back into bed, and replaced it with a sack of tanner's bark over which the scanty mourners squeezed their tears.

William Burke was short and spry, adept at the jig, nimble-witted, and affable. William Hare had a skew face, left eye higher than right, large thick-lipped mouth, hollow cheeks, and laughed a lot. His tumbledown two-story house was crammed with beds (threepence a night, but you had to share with two others). Privacy lay in a small back room overlooking a pigsty. Both men had come from Ireland to work on the Union Canal being dug between Edinburgh and Glasgow.

The pair were appalled at the profligacy of letting rot underground something worth £7.10s—particularly as the doctor cordially implied he would be glad to see them with more. Where from? Unfortunately, the dead did not hang on every tree. Retailers Burke and Hare like Marks and Spencer and Saks Fifth Avenue decided to create their own products.

A miller in Hare's house was ill of the fever, annoyingly repelling customers. They held a pillow over his face. He was likely to die anyway. He fetched £10. On February 11, 1828, they invited into the room over the pigsty an old beggarwoman called Abigail, filled her with whisky, did it by hand, nailed her in a tea-chest and delivered her to Dr. Knox, who was delighted with her freshness. The split was set at £4 to Burke, £5 to Hare and £1 to Mrs. Hare for ancillary duties. It was she who shortly filled a pair of stray women with whisky, Hare did one, Burke the other.

On April 9, an 18-year-old tart, Mary Patterson, was released from a night in the Canongate watch house. She met Burke in a tavern, he filled her up with rum and bitters, took her home for breakfast (tea, bread, eggs, Finnan haddies), and poured her a bottle of whisky. She passed out, got done before lunch, was delivered in the afternoon, made £8 (prices were seasonal, less in summer).

Mary Patterson died with tuppence-ha'penny irremovably tight in her hand (cadaveric spasm, occurs before rigor mortis). As the pair had crossed High School Yards with the sack, the boys all jeered they were carrying a corpse. This voluptuous conscript to their instructors provided a nasty turn for several students and Knox's assistant Mr. Fergusson (later Sir William Fergusson, Bt, Sergeant-Surgeon to Queen Victoria), who had known her professionally in Canongate. One Velazquez of the scalpel sketched Mary as a defunct Rokeby Venus. She would have been dissected to bits within four hours of death, but Dr. Knox wanted to save her for his lecture on female musculature and kept her in a barrel of whisky three months.

Burke was otherwise a cobbler. An old cinder-gatherer called Effie brought him some scraps of leather, was stupified with whisky, made £10. Early one morning, Burke relieved two policemen of a drunk woman being dragged to the West Port watch house, said he knew her lodgings, took her home, got £10 for her.

June came, cleansing breezes blowing from the Forth, chimneys reeking sparsely into the pale blue sky, the castle high on its mound as threatening as a thundercloud. An Irishwoman with her twelve-year-old grandson arrived from Glasgow searching for friends, was kindly directed by Burke, invited home, filled with whisky, done. The child was a damnable difficulty. They could take him out and lose him, but he might return with a policeman. Next day he was asking tearfully after grandma, Burke broke his back. They had to use a herring-barrel for the pair of them. In the Mealmarket, Hare's horse collapsed between the shafts of his cart, a crowd gathered, they urgently sent to Dr. Knox for a porter with a handcart. They got £16 for the pair, the horse went to the knacker's.

On the anniversary of the Battle of Bannockburn, Mrs. Hare urged Burke to turn his live-in love Helen McDougall into stock-in-trade, but he took her on holiday to Falkirk instead. Hare meanwhile made £8 on his account, causing a quarrel that moved Burke to a basement down the lane, sleeping on straw. Like discordant Gilbert and Sullivan, their prosperity depended on an irksome partnership. They did for Helen's distant cousin Ann (Burke fastidiously had Hare perform the stifling). Dr. Knox thought the pair justified a trunk for further supplies (see Chapter 28, Doctor Death).

Next, their charwoman Mrs. Hostler (£8), ninepence-ha'-penny gripped in her dead hand. Then Mrs. Haldane and her daughter Peggy (tarts). Then eighteen-year-old Daft Jamie, imbecile well known to Edinburgh and his dissectors (Knox ordered the head removed first). Jamie had put up a fight, bit Burke, Knox treated him. Finally Mrs. Madge Docherty on All Saints Eve. Two lodgers squealed, the police found her in a tea-chest in the cellar at No. 10 Surgeons' Square. Early on the Sunday morning of November 2, Burke and Hare were arrested. Edinburgh erupted. The *Evening Courant* sold an extra 8,000 copies an issue.

The trial started at ten in the morning of Christmas Eve. The quality of Bench and Bar was there, delighting in pawky, rarefied legal quibble. It continued nonstop until 9:30 on Christmas Day, when the jury found Burke guilty. The judge had ordered the windows kept open, the lawyers wrapping their heads against freezing drafts in gowns and colored handkerchiefs. His only expressed doubts were whether Burke's body should be exhibited in chains or his skeleton preserved as a minatory momento. Hare had spared himself a dreadful night by turning King's evidence.

Burke was hanged in the Lawnmarket at 8:15 on the depressingly wet morning of Wednesday, January 18, 1829, before 25,000 people, including Sir Walter Scott. A view from a window cost 5s to £1. The hangman's entourage fought for fragments of the rope. He was taken for dissection to Professor Monro, who next day lectured on his brain (unusually soft). On Friday the public were admitted, 30,000 all day past the black marble slab. His remaining bits were pickled in barrels for future reference. I encountered his scrotum at a delightful dinner of the Royal College of Surgeons of Edinburgh.

As Burke fell the cry rose, "Hang Knox!" The mob burnt his effigy, stormed his house, broke his windows. He was smuggled away cloaked, armed with sword, pistols, and skean-dhu, guarded by police. Knox was baffled at the populace implicating him in 16 murders. A gentleman engrossed in the intellectual intricacies of the human frame frets not over the origin of the anonymous example before him—no more than he would concern himself whether the fine pheasant bought from a villager for his dinner might be poached. Knox was vindicated by a committee of Scottish noblemen and gentry appointed by himself. But the students he faced began to dwindle, the animosities to rise. In ten years he was out of Surgeons' Square, in fifteen out of work.

Like Robert Liston, Knox turned his back on his unforgiving countrymen for London. He wrote about whales and practiced obstetrics in Hackney, where he died of apoplexy aged 71. Hare was last seen wandering two miles south of Carlisle across the English border, on Sunday morning, February 8, 1829. Burke lives in the eternal glory of the *Oxford English Dictionary: "To kill secretly by suffocation or strangulation . . . 'hush up,' suppress quietly."*

Burke and Hare bestowed through their influence Lord Warburton's Anatomy Act of 1832. Matters are better regulated now. In Britain, if you wish to leave yourself for medical students, fill in form AA1. The authorities concerned send their own hearse and coffin, and pay for your eventual fragmented funeral.

# 9

## RIEN NE VA PLUS
### Disastrous French Bedside Manner

I often recall to memory an anecdote told by the late Dr. Sutherland of Bath. While in Paris, he attended the L'Hôpital de la Charité. One day he accompanied the physician running through one of the wards to visit the patients, a friar trotting after him with his book in hand to minute down the prescriptions; the doctor stops at a bed, and calls out to the person in it, with the utmost precipitation, *"Toussez-vous? Suez-vous? Allez-vous à la selle?"* Then turning instantly to the friar, *"Purgez le."* *"Monsieur, il est mort,"* replied the friar. *"Diable! Allons!"* said the doctor and galloped on with rapidity.

—*William Cuming (1714-1788)*

# 10

## SCUTARI

### *Miss Nightingale vs. the British Army*

The things they say about Florence Nightingale.

"She was a shocking nurse," affirmed her sister Parthenope, who had felt her relentless touch. She was not a ministering angel but a resolute administrator and ruthless politician. She did not sail for the Crimea with dedicated high-born ladies, but a mixture of agitated nuns and ginny Sarah Gamps.

She was named because her mother happened to be staying at Florence while on the Italian tour, and she could as easily have been called Leghorn. The lamp on her statue in Pall Mall and illuminating the £10 note is wrong. She carried a linen Turkish lamp like a Chinese lantern. The soldiers were supposed to kiss her shadow. I have been in the dark with a nurse and the lamp at Miss Nightingale's St. Thomas's Hospital, and it does not throw light enough to kiss anything.

The Crimean War was a medical disaster because the British Army was still fighting Waterloo, where supplies were a luxury and welfare a fantasy.

The four-towered *Selinie Quicklaci* barracks beside the vast Scutari cemetery—still seen across the Bosphorus like a massive upturned billiard table—was made a hospital by whitewashing the walls. There were no bandages or bedpans, mattresses or mugs, food or fuel. Istanbul, lying far further south than Bournemouth, was assumed in London to be hot.

They had plenty of rats and lice, and 250 soldiers' wives and widows getting drunk and prostituting themselves in the basement. They had some wooden operating tables but chopped them up for firewood. In the bitter November of 1854, Miss Nightingale and 1,050 casualties from the Charge of the Light Brigade arrived simultaneously.

The army doctor in charge of Scutari was across the Black Sea at Balaklava—Dr. John Hall, who forbade chloroform because "the smart of the knife is a powerful stimulant, and it is better to hear a man bawl lustily than to see him sink silently into his grave." The only nurses were soldiers unfit for anything else. Medical stores from home were labelled "Not Urgent," and the *Prince* bringing them sailed first to the Crimea, where she sank in a hurricane.

The wounded packed on the transports from the Crimea to Turkey had abandoned their knapsacks in the summer's forced march on the Alma, possessed only filthy greatcoats as blankets on deck, suffered frostbite, dysentery, typhus, scurvy, and cholera, went overboard dead at a dozen a day. At Scutari, the daily death rate from four miles of patients lining its floors was 45. The stench penetrated the walls. As Bernard Shaw mentioned, "The British soldier can stand up to anything except the British War Office."

Miss Nightingale was crammed into the "Sisters' Tower" (found to contain a dead Russian general), in company with 40 nurses paid 12s a week (double London pay), dressed in hideous uniforms (to repel the men), and allowed to drink gin (in moderation). She could not enter a ward without an army doctor's order. The army preferred to ignore her. The nurses sewed idly. But Miss Nightingale had a way of getting her way. "I MUST remember God is not my private secretary," she once wrote a note to herself.

Florence Nightingale had a rich, idle father, a fashionable matchmaking mother, and a flower-arranging sister. She was 34 and had confessed the nursing urge ten years before to Julia Ward Howe, the American suffragist. Her family was perplexed and disgusted. A nurse was lower socially than the maid who emptied their slop buckets. The Institution for the Care of Sick Gentlewomen in Distressed Circumstances in Harley Street timorously appointed her superintendent there, driving her mother to sal volatile, her sister to bed for a week, and her father to the Atheneum Club.

Within months she installed windlass dumbwaiters for the food, piped hot water, and a bleeping system with bells, banned the crinoline, killed the vermin, fired the house-surgeon, cut up the worn slipcovers for dishcloths, bulk-ordered the groceries from Fortnum and Mason's, made her own jam at tuppence a pot, took a patients' library subscription at Mudie's, and reduced the daily cost of each inmate from 1s 10d to 1s. She would have been equally efficient running Dartmoor Prison and probably as happy.

The Sick Gentlewomen were valuable guinea pigs for the sick soldier. Next year at Scutari she swabbed the wards, emptied the overflowing latrine-tubs, scoured the drains (producing 2 dead horses, 24 assorted animals and 556 handcarts of rubbish), stuffed straw in bags for beds, found cauldrons to heat the water, set the soldiers' wives scrubbing and washing, raided the quartermaster's stores, broke all regulations, and defied everybody, knowing she could never be court-marshalled.

Miss Nightingale had two priceless allies. William Howard Russell's chilling dispatches had crystalized national fury. His *Times* raised £30,000 for her use in the bazaars of Constantinople. She bought knives and forks, soap and towels, food and drink, bedding and clothing—you were nursed in what you were wounded in. The British ambassador was baffled at her rejecting his suggestion of using the money to raise British prestige by erecting a Protestant church.

M. Alexis Soyer, famous chef of the Reform Club, as exuberantly French as only one who lived all his life in London could be left for Scutari on an impulse over scalloped oysters and port in Drury Lane. He redeployed the kitchens and drilled the cooks, applied intelligence and flavoring to the salt meat, sheep heads, cow heels and offal, turned the inedible into the desirable. The men cheered him in the wards. "Though admittedly it has no nourishing qualities, there is nothing yet discovered which is substitute to the English for . . ." Ah! Miss Nightingale! Your genius for essentials! ". . . his cup of tea."

"The Bird" claimed justly to have started nursing the British army, then clothing it, feeding it, writing its letters home, making its wills, and burying a good proportion of it. "Nursing is the least of the functions into which I have been forced." She had plenty of dirty women to do the dirty work.

Miss Nightingale presided that winter at 2,000 deathbeds. The mortality fell to 5 percent in spring. The last patient left in summer the following year. She had been at war for 632 days and came home with a reputation that would last her all her life. She went to bed for 50 years. From her Mayfair couch she reorganized the Army Medical Department, sanitated portions of India, founded her nurses' training school, wrote *Notes on Nursing* and *Suggestions for Thought to the Searchers after Truth among the Artizans of England,* to which Mr. John Stuart Mill was most kind. Cabinet ministers, generals, viceroys entered her bedroom beseeching advice, Master of Balliol Jowett that she should marry him. It was an age when women's liberation meant going without stays. They gave her the Order of Merit, and she died, aged 90.

Miss Nightingale revolutionized nursing by making a chambermaid's work an occupation for gentlewomen. Her system was so sound that her antiseptic ghost haunts every sickbed. Wherever you are ill, you are still nursed by Florence Nightingale.

She was a woman of whom her country is rightly proud, because she could not possibly have come from any other.

# 11

## CLUBROOM DOCTOR
### *Disastrous Negligence (60 Percent)*

Sir Samuel Garth, coming to the Kit Kat club one night, declared he must soon be gone, having many patients to attend; but some good wine being produced he forgot them. Sir Richard Steele was of the party and reminded him of the visits he had to pay, when Garth immediately pulled out his list, which amounted to fifteen, and said: "It's no great matter whether I see them tonight or not, for nine of them have such bad constitutions that all the physicians in the world can't save them, and the other six have such good constitutions that all the physicians in the world can't kill them."

—*John Timbs (1801-1875)*

# Part Three

# LET ALL YE
# WHO ENTER HERE . . .

# 12

## DISASTROUS MOTHERHOOD
### *Tales from the Vienna Wards*

The Autocrat of the Breakfast Table was superbly dictatorial on February 13, 1843:

> A physician holding himself in readiness to attend cases of midwifery should never take any active part in the postmortem examination of cases of puerperal fever.
>
> If a physician is present at such autopsies, he should use thorough ablution, change every article of dress, and allow twenty-four hours or more to elapse before attending to any case of midwifery. It may be well to extend the same caution to cases of simple peritonitis.
>
> On the occurrence of a single case of puerperal fever in his practice, the physician is bound to consider the next female he attends in labor, unless some weeks at least have elapsed, as in danger of being infected by him . . . the time has come when the existence of a private pestilence in the sphere of a single physician, should be looked upon not as a misfortune but a crime.

Dr. Oliver Wendell Holmes was addressing the Boston Society for Medical Improvement. His suggested simple improvement of washing the hands in chloride of lime before delivering a child outraged obstetricians, particularly in Philadelphia.

Countered the autocrat, "Medical logic does not appear to be taught or practiced in our schools."

Surgeons operated in blood-stiffened frock coats—the stiffer the coat the prouder the busy surgeon—hanging on pegs at the theater door with *boutonnières* of waxed hemp stitches. Pus was as inseparable from surgery as blood. The yellow ooze from every wound was cheerfully classified as "laudable pus." "Sanious pus" was unwelcome, and "ichorous pus" the stinking herald of cadaverous putrefaction.

Cleanliness was next to prudishness. "There was no object in being clean," later wrote Sir Frederick "Elephant Man" Treves. "Indeed, cleanliness was out of place. It was considered to be finicking and affected. An executioner might as well manicure his nails before chopping off a head."

Puerperal fever terrorized the week after labor. The mother suddenly felt ill, shook with rigors. The lochia discharging from her vagina turned stinking and bloody. Peritonitis developed, thrombosis in the legs, abcesses in the breasts, infection of the lungs and brain, bleeding into the skin, stupor, and death. Hippocrates had marked it a disease generally fatal and mysteriously transmitted.

In 1846, Ignaz Philipp Semmelweis was appointed assistant in the First Obstetric Clinic at the *Allgemeine Krankenhaus,* Vienna. He was short, bald, elegantly mustached, sensitive, excitable, aged 28, Hungarian. The vast General Hospital was built by Empress Maria Theresa, among her bounties to her motley people after the Peace of Paris ended the Seven Years' War in 1763.

It encompassed the biggest lying-in hospital in the world. This was divided into the First Clinic, five wards for teaching medical students, and the adjoining Second Clinic, another five for teaching midwives. The mortality from puerperal fever in the First was three times that in the Second.

This was all around Vienna. Weeping women implored their confinement in the Second Clinic. The gloom of childbirth in the First was deepened by its remoteness from the hospital chapel— the last sacrament was borne directly to the dying in the Second Clinic, but to reach the sickroom of the First, robed priests needed to troop through all five wards behind their tolling bell. Elsewhere in the hospital once a day sufficed, but 24 hours is a long time in puerperal fever, and the doomful parade became an all-too familiar sight.

Semmelweis could pick only one path down the mortality gradient. It led the First Clinic's students to perform vaginal examinations direct from the dissecting-room, casually washing their fingers in between. The midwives of the Second Clinic took a cleaner journey to work.

On March 20, 1847, Semmelweis's colleague, Jacobus Kolletschka, Professor of Medical Jurisprudence, died after his finger was wounded by a student while together they cut up a corpse. The professor's riven body in the postmortem room inspired Semmelweis to conclude that the disease that killed the professor and countless new mothers was the same.

> Semmelweis wrote: Day and night the vision of Kolletschka's malady haunted me. It was not the wound, but the wound rendered unclean by cadaveric material, which had produced the fatal result. . . . I must therefore put this question to myself; did then the individuals whom I have seen die from an identical disease also have cadaveric matter carried into the vascular system? To this question I must answer, Yes!

Every mother had a wound. It was the raw womb that had shed its placenta in the afterbirth.

He ordered his students to wash their hands in chloride of lime. The mortality in the First Clinic fell from 18 to one percent. Semmelweis bettered Oliver Wendel Holmes, in perceiving puerperal fever a poisoning of the blood. The European doctors bettered the American ones in bigotry. Semmelweis retired to Budapest.

On July 31, 1865, Semmelweis's friend Ferdinant Hebra found some pretext of enticing him from his wife and infant to the local madhouse. The sadly necessary intention was to keep the now mentally unbalanced physician there. The asylum doctor noticed a small wound on a right finger, incurred at Semmelweis's last operation. It turned gangrenous, ate into the finger-joint, infection spread up the arm, and abcesses formed in the lungs. Semmelweiss died on August 13 from the equivalent of puerperal fever.

The disease is no longer in the index of obstetrical textbooks.

# 13

## DESIGN FOR LIVING

### *Bricks and Mortality*

"It may seem a strange principle to enunciate as the very first requirement in a Hospital . . ." Florence Nightingale had a nose for the elusive obvious ". . . that it should do the sick no harm."

She meant architecturally, not clinically.

There was an awesome row in 1856. The army was building a hospital in Hampshire, to look as impressive upon Southampton Water as the Scutari *Selinie Quicklaci* upon the Bosporus. Miss Nightingale damned it from watercloset to weathercock.

A Royal Commission tentatively asked if she had devoted attention to hospital design. "Yes," Miss Nightingale crisply told them, "for thirteen years I have visited all the hospitals in London, Dublin, and Edinburgh, many county hospitals, some of the naval and military hospitals in England, all the hospitals in Paris and the Institution of Protestant Deaconesses at Kaiserwerth on the Rhine, the hospitals at Berlin and many others in Germany, at Lyons, Rome, Alexandria, Constantinople, Brussels, also the war hospitals of the French and the Sardinians."

Miss Nightingale knew the best saucepans for the kitchen, the best books for the library, the best color for the walls (pale pink). And she had written *A Treatise on Sinks*.

A new army hospital was a brick block pierced by corridors as long as rifle-shots. Miss Nightingale wanted a row of pavilions, so that the ward air might not mix and contaminate. Like Semmelweis, she countered the activities of germs long before they clinically existed. Her pavilioned shrine of St. Thomas's Hospital still edifies Members of Parliament taking tea across the Thames on their terrace.

The Victorian Secretary at War rebuffed her. He could hardly demolish the half-built walls, and at a cost of £70,000. Miss Nightingale spent the weekend with Prime Minister Lord Palmerston. He decided he would rather pay to throw it brick by brick into Southampton Water.

Nobody dared build a hospital in the British Empire without consulting Florence Nightingale. She had never been shipped somewheres east of Suez, but she knew where to look it up. If she ineffectively raged at the viceroy for not opening Indian hospital windows in the burning sun which would have dissipated the precious cool of night, she did it lying in bed all day in Mayfair.

The modern sick are more likely to be harmed by the hospital tumbling about their ears, the newer the building the riskier. The British Department of Health has a £30m a year bill for hospital defects. The General Hospital at Bangor in Wales needed urgent redesign when someone noticed the pathology department drains went through the kitchen. At the new University Hospital in Cardiff, the roof tiles were flaking like dandruff. The newer Monyhull Geriatric Unit in Birmingham cost £360,000 to build, then £88,000 to put right. Other hospitals needed intensive care for incipient collapse at Walsall, Basingstoke, Rhyl, North Ayrshire, and Glasgow. The nationwide epidemic struck the world-famous Great Ormond Street Hospital for Children in London. Its new cardiac unit (£7½m) was evacuated within a year when found to incorporate within its shoddy structural supports a virtual do-it-yourself earthquake.

The biggest constructional disaster was St. George's Hospital at Hyde Park Corner, perfect site for a luxury hotel, views into Buckingham Palace. The Tory Government in 1982 sold it back to the Duke of Westminster for the £23,700 they paid in 1906. It was in the contract. The Labour spokeswoman described the deal as "extraordinary." This was the best left-wing British understatement since Clement Attlee used no words when one would do.

# 14

## CATASTROPHE

### *Heartbreaking Hospital Hazard*

The British are ruthlessly businesslike. When Queen Victoria sought the 82-year-old Duke of Wellington's counsel on sparrows infesting the crystal domes of the 1851 Great Exhibition, he replied instantly, "Sparrowhawks, ma'am." (They worked.)

In 1982, engineers at the North Middlesex Hospital, Edmonton, London, asked advice from the Minister of Health about a feral colony of 40 cats fouling the heating ducts with droppings and fleas. "Shoot 'em!" he directed.

In the quiet of a Sunday afternoon, a pest control man slipped into the hospital and stealthily started stalking pussies. A shot rang out. The sniper's fate was in the papers.

"We heard the shooting about 5 P.M.," one eyewitness said. "We saw a man with a rifle. One of the women tried to take his gun away."

"While my man was doing his duty," the pest boss complained angrily, "three women came out using very bad language. One of them had a long pole with a nail at the end, and they hit his rifle."

The British are euphorically sentimental over small animals. The stray cats of Edmonton—a district with little to spare after feeding itself—sprang through the hospital windows to enjoy central heating, kitchen scraps, and the affection of the hospital workers, all three at the expense of the impoverished National

Health Service. A stranger going around shooting them was barely less horrendous than one going around to shoot the geriatric patients.

Six cats were bagged in that Sunday shoot-out. One escaped, wounded with a .22 bullet; the domestic staff, in the hope of finding and succoring it, diverted itself all week.

"Our priority is the care of patients and how to protect them from cats climbing in through windows," the Ministry of Health vindicated itself stiffly. CAT—the Cat Action Trust—suggested neutering, instead. It is better to be castrated than catsmeat.

"Experience has shown that if you remove one set of cats," explained the CAT lady, "a vacuum is created that is immediately filled by others. A stable neutered colony not only does not multiply but keeps new cats away." As CAT estimates a million feral cats in Britain, the sterilizers are going to be more outrageously overworked than the National Health Service doctors.

The Duke of Wellington would have suggested putting in ferrets.

# 15

## RUDE AWAKENING

### *Frozen Assets*

A clammy summer night in the accident department. Young man in T-shirt and jeans lies screened on a couch. He was brought in by ambulance, deeply unconscious.

The intern is new, young, female, pretty, clever. She doubts the diagnosis. He responds as a healthy person would to tests. She wonders if he's shamming. Could it be that he's really wide awake? People *do* behave so oddly in hospitals.

Doctor and nurse confer. "Why not," suggests the nurse sensibly, "spray his genitals with ethyl chloride? *That* will show pretty smartly if he's swinging the lead."

Excellent idea!

Ethyl chloride is a colorless liquid, highly volatile, once popular as a rough-and-ready local anesthetic. Instant evaporation when sprayed on the skin produces a frozen numbness, enough for operations like opening abcesses, removing small warts, piercing ears.

Doctor and nurse unzip their patient's fly, retract his Y-fronts, take aim, spray. The action is spectacular. A fine, frosty film forms on the skin, like the bloom on deep-frozen meatballs.

Instant effect.

Patient jumps up, pulls together clothes, storms from hospital.

Case not concluded. A hot letter complains of his privates getting a cold shower. Disastrous litigation avoided by hospital diplomatically insisting that he had after all suffered no harm in the two ladies' hands.

He agreed.

A lot of men might quite like it.

# Part Four

# GERM WARFARE

# 16

## TYPHOID MARY

### *Death on a Plate*

"The cook was a good cook, as cooks go; and as cooks go she went," Saki wrote in 1904. Mary Mallon was then traversing the spacious, moneyed houses of New York State. She had eight jobs in seven years. Among seven families, her tenure coincided with a nasty outbreak of typhoid fever.

At Mamaroneck in 1900, a young man who came to stay in September got typhoid ten days later. Mary spent 1901 in New York City. The household laundress died of typhoid in Roosevelt Hospital just before Christmas. The next summer took her to Dark Harbor, Maine, into a lawyer's household of eight—seven down with typhoid in a fortnight. The lawyer was immune from an earlier attack. Mary devoted herself to the sick so unsparingly he gave her an extra $50.

She moved in 1904 to Sands Point, Long Island. Typhoid broke out a week later, four cases out of ten, all domestics. The New York City Health Department decided there was something mysteriously noxious about the servants' quarters. Typhoid exploded a week after Mary's arrival at Oyster Bay on Long Island Sound in 1909 (six out of ten, three family, three servants). While Colonel Gorgas was boasting he had freed Panama from yellow fever, New York City suffered that year 3,467 cases of typhoid with 639 deaths.

The disease seldom seeped from the city into Oyster Bay. Dr. George A. Soper hurried from New York, busied himself with the milk, the water, the family fare, the well and the cesspool, the cistern and the privy, the manure spread on the lawn. What did they like most to eat? Clams. Clams! Typhoid grenades. For sure, it was the fault of that old Indian woman who lived on the beach and peddled clams at the back door.

Typhoid is patchy inflammation of the small intestine, which coils in the abdomen like an inflated condom six feet long. The patient develops a steadily rising fever, a fleeting rash, bellyache, cough, greenish diarrhea (the "staircase temperature, rose spots, and pea-soup stools" of florid Edwardian physicians). Today it is cured with the antibiotic chloramphenicol. In the time of Typhoid Mary, like most illnesses you either got better or died according to your luck.

The germs have long hairlike flagellae and can scuttle about. A tiny dose can bring a widespread epidemic, through water, food, milk, flies. These are contaminated by the feces of a carrier who has recovered from the disease, perhaps an attack too mild to identify. In the 1900s, this conception of apparently healthy carriers first explained the mysterious scattering of typhoid epidemics. One typhoid patient in twenty continues excreting live bacteria for a year. Some, intermittently for life. These are nearly all women.

Luckily for the Indian's trade, nobody in the Oyster Bay house had eaten clams for six weeks, well outside the incubation period. What else did they enjoy? asked Dr. Soper. The cook's ice cream was delicious. Oh, not the present cook. The one who left suddenly, three weeks after the typhoid started.

Dr. Soper found the cook six months later. He traced her through Tuxedo, N.Y. (one case) to Park Avenue (two servants suffering typhoid, the daughter of the house dead with it).

Mary Mallon was 40, unmarried, an immigrant from Northern Ireland. She had thick graying hair, round steel-rimmed glasses, straight full eyebrows, a placid face with a mouth turned down at the corners. Her fat figure was a good reference. She was shy, surly, sullen, and secretive.

They met in the kitchen. Dr. Soper tactfully suggested some connection between these sickly visitations and her floury fingers. She attacked him with a cleaver. He bolted and hastened to the New York Health Commissioner, who called the police. Mary gave them the slip. As they were leaving a policeman spotted a scrap of striped skirt caught in a neighboring privy door. They piled ashcans against it and called on her to surrender. She came out fighting. Biting, screaming, kicking, she was removed in an ambulance, an inspector from the City Health Department sitting on her chest.

They took Mary to the Riverside Hospital for communicable diseases on North Brother Island, in the East River off the Bronx, 13 acres facing Rikers Island jail. The press fed on her with relish. Mary was drawn as a comicstrip witch, dropping skulls into the pot, sizzling on the stove typhoid bacilli the size of frankfurters. The public was hysterical. How many malevolent Marys were there, murdering New Yorkers without the inconvenience of breaking the law?

Dr. Soper took a swab from her stools, incubated it, and looked down his microscope. Teeming with typhoid bacilli. He explained patiently she had a fatal disease—for other people. Typhoid germs were breeding in her gallbladder as cosily as bees in a hive. The cure was straightforward—removal of gallbladder.

Mary had no spark of the dazzling altruism that blinded the fabled Pole afflicted with the evil eye, who put out his sight lest he harm his children. She refused. Quite rightly, too. A cholecystectomy in 1907 was as uninviting as a heart transplant today. Dr. Soper suggested the less painful alternative of abandoning cooking. She objected that cooking was her livelihood, a skill affording her pride and delight. They kept her in Riverside for three years.

Mary was a morose prisoner-patient, angry, rebellious, threatening, certain she was the victim of a doctors' plot. She refused to admit, perhaps even to believe, that she was a typhoid carrier. She worked as a hospital laundress, winning her release in 1910 with a promise to stay at the scrub board instead of the stove, and to report tri-monthly to the Health Department.

She disappeared. She became Mrs. Brown, the cook. She was not like a jailbird heartlessly resuming dangerous crime as a familiar living. She was expressing her independence, her defiance, her resentment toward fellow humans who fearfully accused her of casting spells.

For five years Mary worked unsuspected in the kitchens of New York. Typhoid cases followed her as surely as crows carrion. The disease was too commonplace for anxious speculation of each source. In 1915 a serious epidemic affected the staff of the Sloane Hospital for Women, New York (25 cases, two deaths). The kitchenmaids called the cook "Typhoid Mary" for a joke. She fled. When the police found her working on Long Island, she went quietly.

Mary returned to North Brother Island. She had earned herself the sentence of quarantine for life. The Health Department could never risk freeing again the newspapers' ghoul of the griddle. Even embittered typhoid carriers mellow with age. Gradually Mary accepted possessing the guiltless danger of a hungry tiger at large. She went over to the enemy, working as a Riverside laboratory technician. New York, too, became kindlier. In 1923 the city built her a cottage beside the hospital, where she gave tea parties.

Mary had a stroke on Christmas Day 1932. She never walked again. Riverside cared for her tenderly. She got religion. She never spoke of family or birthplace. Typhoid was an unmentionable subject. She died on November 11, 1938, of bronchopneumonia complicating chronic nephritis and myocarditis, excreting typhoid to the last.

Her official score was 53 cases and three deaths. Her unattributed ones must have been vastly more. Hers was probably the 1903 epidemic of 1,400 cases at Ithaca in upstate New York.

Mary Mallon was America's first named typhoid carrier. When she died, 300 were known in New York, all prevented from working with food or water. The title of "New York Carrier No. 1" escaped her. When there were sufficient to warrant a list, Mary came alphabetically No. 36.

Only nine people went to her funeral. Every doctor in the world knows her name.

# 17

## ST. ANTHONY'S FIRE

### *Bakehouse Disaster*

On August 15, 1951, the Provencal village of Pont Saint Esprit went mad.

One in twenty of its 4,000 inhabitants were seized with delirium and hallucinations, ran wild in the streets, writhed and screamed in their beds, suffered nausea, colic, vomiting, insomnia, and burning sensations, particularly in the anus. Four died.

It was St. Anthony's fire, *ignis sacer, mal des ardents,* scourge of the medieval peasantry. You feel you are being burned at the stake. Your fingers and toes, hands and feet drop off. If doubly unlucky, you have convulsions (it depends on your level of vitamin A).

The cause is bread milled from "smutty" rye infected with ergot fungus (*Claviceps purpurea*), as anyone would tell you in the seventeenth century. The ergot grows purple spurs on the ears of rye, particularly after a wet sowing and a wet summer.

Thucydides' Plague of Athens was really ergot poisoning. It was uninfectious—no other Athenian cities got it. The symptoms were too varied for any single disease. The naval expedition to Laconia suffered after loading supplies there. The cause was damaged crops salvaged from Attica.

The English had little taste for rye bread and little ergotism, apart from *A Singular Calamity, Which Suddenly Happened to a poor Family of this Parish, Of which Six Persons lost their Feet by a Mortification not to be accounted for,* perpetuated by a 1762 tablet in Wattisham village church, Suffolk.

Ergot contains an LSD-like chemical found also in morning glory seeds, the everyday hallucinogen of the Aztecs. As drugs account for peculiar behavior today, so bread in the middle ages. The eleven girl accusers in the Salem witchcraft trials of 1692— who suffered "distempers" of odd speech, postures, and gestures, and fits—may have achieved the hanging of 19 fellow-creatures, and the pressing to death of another, while high on ergot.

Perhaps Aldous Huxley's 17 orgiastic nuns possessed by the devils of Loudun—whose *furor uterinus* had priest Grandier truly burnt at the stake—defeated their energetic exorcists because they were only coming through the rye.

# 18

## LUCKLESS LÜBECK

### *Vaccine Backfires*

"My brother was an invalid," recounted Anthony Trollope, "and the horrid word, which of all words was, for some years after, the most dreadful to us, had been pronounced. . . . My younger sister Emily, with that false-tongued hope which knows the truth but will lie lest the heart should faint, had been called delicate, but only delicate, was now ill. Of course she was doomed."

The unspeakable word today is cancer. In 1834 it was consumption. Trollope's brother Henry was dead by Christmas, Emily two years later at 18, four of his children died from it between 12 and 33. His contemporary Dickens named it the disease that "medicine never cured, wealth never warded off."

"Captain of all these men of death that came against him to take him away," wrote John Bunyan about Mr. Badman, "was the Consumption, for it was that that brought him down to the grave." (Tuberculosis is the most literary of diseases.)

The Captain was most active in his work from the end of the eighteenth century to the middle of the next. Napoleon ravaged Europe, but tuberculosis filled a quarter of its graves. In the Eastern States, it killed 5 in 1,000 Americans, 130 in 1,000 if they happened to be in jail (and white, the black rates were worse). Quaker physician Thomas Young confessed consumption "so fatal as to deter practitioners from attempting a cure."

Familiar names are carved on the Captain's memorial. Charlotte and Emily Brontë, coughing over each other behind closed windows amid the Yorkshire moors, their two sisters already dead. Robert Louis Stevenson hopelessly seeking health in Samoa, George Orwell turning as desperately to Scotland, D. H. Lawrence to Nice, the *Yellow Book's* Aubrey Beardsley to Menton. Dr. Anton Chekhov at 44, Edgar Allen Poe and Franz Kafka at 40. Raphael, Watteau, and Modigliani. Paganini, Purcell, Chopin, and Mozart. Mimi and Louis Dubedat on stage.

"I know the colour of that blood," cried Dr. John Keats the first time he spat it. "It is arterial blood, I cannot be deceived in that colour. That drop of blood is my death warrant—I must die."

Lying fevered and wasting in his little square room by the Spanish Steps in Rome, Keats implored his devoted friend, the painter Joseph Severn, "You must not look at me in my dying gasp, nor breathe my passing breath." Few were so worried that consumption might be catching. Its prevalence masked its infectivity. It seemed an affliction as natural as death itself.

The Verona physician Hieronymous Frascastorius suspected in 1546 that it was contagious. In England two hundred years later, Dr. Benjamin Martin's *New Theory of Consumption* depicted animalculae fretting and gnawing in stomach, liver, and lungs. Professor Rudolf Virchow of Berlin—whose microscope magnified Sir Morell Mackenzie's bungles with the crown prince's larynx—thought tuberculosis invaded the body with deadly bundles of cells, like cancer.

Robert Koch was a Rhineland country doctor, who, together with Louis Pasteur, became to germs what Copernicus and Galileo were to the stars. In 1882 he found the cause of tuberculosis, a slender bacillus that grasped a crimson stain too firmly for decolorization with acids—the "acid-fast" bacillus. Many physicians retained their clinical ideas as forcefully. Germs remained German fancies, while death rose from the widespread habit of spitting on the floor.

The cause was found, the cure yearned for. In 1890 Koch was cascaded with honors for discovering it—"tuberculin," a glycerine extract of the bacillus. It was a false claim, the only taint in a career of pure benefaction. The White Plague diminished as the century extended, through better feeding and housing. Dr. S.

Adolphus Knopf of Philadelphia recognized in 1901, "To combat consumption successfully requires the combined action of a wise government, well-trained physicians, and an intelligent people." Applied to diseases now filling the Captain's stealthy boots, the idea could do us a lot of good.

In 1922, Drs. Calmette and Guérin vaccinated a child with attenuated cow TB, producing immunity to the human disease. There was not even a painful injection, you swallowed it. Every parent wanted so sure, so safe a way of saving his family. And if tuberculosis could be prevented in individuals, surely it could be eliminated from the world?

In the spring of 1930, some children given Bacille Calmette-Guérin in the German port of Lübeck became ill, one died. It caused no stir. Children were always being ill that time of year. Then another 14 died. Prophylaxis with "BCG" stopped. Of 249 children vaccinated between February 24 and April 25, 73 were dead by autumn. Those dosed in the ten days of mid-March and the end of April suffered nine-tenths of the deaths.

No secret virulence could have surged in the harmless culture of germs supplied by the Institute Pasteur in Paris. A hundred children vaccinated from the same batch across the Baltic at Riga were fine. The Minister of the Interior had interested himself when the dead children reached 52. For a politician to ride a tragedy, he fires criminal charges from the saddle. The hospital, the children's clinic, and four laboratory directors were accused of manslaughter.

The police found that the stock of deadly doses and the original germs from Paris had mysteriously been destroyed. Doctors gossiped about a virulent vial of human TB germs from Kiel, which had lost its label in the same Lübeck laboratory. Inquisitive Dr. Ludwig Lange found a forgotten ampule of the vanished vaccine and grew its bacilli in bacteriologists' nutritive soup. A green tinge developed, unusual with BCG germs. He tried growing the Kiel germs. They produced green, too. He grew germs taken from the victims' corpses. Green as well.

The coincidence suggested that an unknown patient in Kiel had fatally infected 73 children in Lübeck. The murderous muddle could not be proved. The hospital, the clinic, and the laboratory directors were cleared after a long trial. The disaster was forgotten. Anyway, people were distracted that year by Hitler declaring himself ready to capture the soul of Germany.

In 1930, 12 youngsters died among 559 vaccinated with BCG at Ujpest, Hungary, and one from 10 at Santiago. The vaccine is today given medical students and nurses, and advised for susceptible children. The inoffensive, unconsidered vole, a small rodent that looks much like a fat mouse, has scampered to man's aid. The tuberculosis bacillus that kills voles bestows human immunity, though innocuous to man without the labor of its attenuation.

No longer "Youth grows pale, and spectre thin, and dies." For near a century, youth fought the fell Captain on the battlefields of Davos, Montreux, St. Moritz, living languorously up in the mountains in the guaranteed Swiss air. Dr. Edward Livingstone Trudeau—who saw a doctor's duty "to cure sometimes, to relieve often, to comfort always"—founded a sanatorium in 1882 at Saranac Lake in the Adirondacks. He had developed TB himself, after walking one night the length of New York from Central Park to the Battery in 47 minutes for a bet.

The conjunction of character and circumstance in sanatoria was irresistible to Thomas Mann and Dr. Somerset Maugham (a casualty), particularly as the fever made the victims sexy. The antibiotic streptomycin overcame tuberculosis in the 1950s. It also knocked the bottom out of the Swiss sanatorium market. They became hotels advertising their deep, airy, sunny balconies. I wonder how many people died on them.

# 19

## BITTER VICTORY

### *Spanish Flu*

At the eleventh hour, the eleventh day in the eleventh month, the killing stopped. The world rejoiced, the gods laughed.

The Great War killed 8,538,313 military personnel, 12.5 percent of the 65,038,810 mobilized. The influenza pandemic of 1918 killed 0.5 percent of the entire population of the United States and of England, 3 percent of Sierra Leone's, 25 percent of Samoa's and 60 percent of the Eskimos in Nome, Alaska. In six weeks it killed 3.1 percent of U.S. recruits at Camp Sherman. Five million from India died, the corpses needed removing from trains on arrival. Liners docked with 5 percent fewer passengers than embarked.

The big American push on the Meuse-Argonne front was checked by 70,000 flu casualties. So was Ludendorff's last fling on the Somme. Woodrow Wilson got it, also Lloyd George, Clemenceau, German prime minister Prince Max, and Colonel House.

Nature is a more efficient murderer than man. The war needed four years, the flu barely one. It killed 25,000,000, 3 percent of all cases, our worst plague. A fifth of the global population caught it, it left serological fingerprints on many more who nursed subclinical attacks.

Flu fatalities usually lie in infancy and senility. This epidemic mocked the war by slaughtering the 20–40 age group. Influenza was the tiger, pneumonia the jackal for its unkilled prey. Antibiotics lay as far ahead as Chancellor Hitler.

Where had it come from? The milder first wave started in U.S. military camps during the spring of 1918, to be transported with the troops to France. Thence to Spain, where the epidemic was so violent the disease found its name. There was influenza that spring in China, and Chinese laborers mingled with men from everywhere, crowded into Europe, coughing over each other.

A deadlier wave broke in the autumn, perhaps starting at Ashkhabad in southern Russia, crossing the Iranian border for an outbreak at Mashhad, in the corner against Afghanistan. That August, HMS *Africa* had sailed from Sierra Leone, losing 7 percent of her crew before reaching the English Channel. Like a malign Puck, infection girdled the earth with simultaneous outbreaks in the ports of Freetown, Brest, and Boston. In the U.S., it killed more new immigrants from rural Italy, Russia, Austria, and Poland than from crowded Britain and Germany.

As Boccaccio said of an earlier scourge, "How many valiant men, how many fair ladies, breakfasted with their kinsfolk and that same night supped with their ancestors in the other world." People eyed each other with keener suspicion than during the war's spy scares. To sneeze was like drawing a knife. "Coughing, Sneezing, or Spitting Will Not Be Permitted in the Theater," said the notices outside. "In case you must Cough or Sneeze, do so in your own handkerchief, and if the Coughing or Sneezing Persists Leave the Theater At Once. GO HOME AND GO TO BED UNTIL YOU ARE WELL. If you have a cold or are coughing and sneezing DO NOT ENTER THIS THEATER."

Hospitals had patients in the corridors. Thousands were inoculated with useless antiflu vaccine. Schools and libraries were closed. Men were advised to stop shaves in barberships. Everyone was advised to wear fresh pajamas, avoid shaking hands, take castor oil. The world wore white cotton masks, like surgeons. In San Francisco they were obligatory, on pain of jail (the police complained they encouraged robbery).

Soldiers prudently dug graves for which there were not yet bodies. There was profiteering in coffins. The Washington, D.C., health commissioner commandeered two railroad cars full of them, which a railwayman tipped him off to be lying in the

Potomac freight yards. He stacked them under police guard, coffin-theft being the crime of the moment.

The visitation lingered everywhere for about six weeks. A less lethal wave came with 1919. By the spring, the flu had gone. Where? Perhaps into swine.

It could come back.

# 20

# THE GREEN MONKEYS

## Revenge in the Rhineland

In August 1967, a cargo of African green monkeys was flown from Entebbe in Uganda to Frankfurt in West Germany. They made a stopover in the African-South American room of the Royal Society for the Prevention of Cruelty to Animals' hostel at Heathrow Airport, London.

The green, yellow, or black-furred vervet monkey *Cercopithecus aethiops* was a regular airline passenger. A quarter-million of them had entered Europe and the United States to participate in laboratory research. Their kidneys were wonderful for growing viruses in test-tubes.

The consignment was booked to Marburg, a university town fifty miles north of Frankfurt, where Luther and Zwingli in 1529 disputed on Transubstantiation. Shortly after the monkeys' arrival, staff at the Behringverke Pharmaceutical Company and at the Paul-Ehrlich Institute in Frankfurt were struck by an illness unknown to man.

They developed sudden fever, headache, vomiting, watery diarrhea, widespread pains. They became covered with tiny bright red spots, with reddening of the scrotum or vulva, and blisters in mouth and throat. The liver enlarged, the sex glands were inflamed, the kidney faltered, the heart softened, the brain swelled. Blood oozed from nose, gums, gut, bladder, even the pricks of syringes. A second batch of patients appeared among the doctors, nurses, and families of the first. Thirty-one people caught it, seven died.

It was an alarming disease, even for the uninfected. Nobody at first knew the cause, the treatment, the chances of recovery, how catching it was, how dangerous. Would it ravage susceptible, over-populated Europe, making the Black Death look like a minor accident?

The original patients had handled the green monkeys, either living, dead, or sliced. What made these monkeys unlike their quarter-million harmless little fellows? The answer came from the British germ warfare center at Porton Down. This is isolated in the most beautiful countryside of southern England. Psychologically, it shares a menacing landscape with atomic power stations and atomic-waste dumps, particularly if viewed from the left.

Porton Down calmed the panic by isolating an unknown virus, unusually long with a hook on the end, resembling a monkey wrench. They could grow it on cells from baby hamster kidneys or from the human foreskin.

The Marburg monkeys were meanwhile traced to the Lake Kyoga region, north of Kampala, all from the same monkey trapper. The disease they carried to Europe was not even a symptomless monkey disease. Doctors proved this by injecting green monkeys with the virus and finding the lot died.

All admittedly hard luck on the monkeys. The sensitive and high-minded, who revolt against such experiments on animals for the benefit of us all, should know their two most powerful allies this century—it was in evidence at a Nürnberg trial—were Adolf Hitler and Hermann Göring.

The Marburg virus probably lives naturally in a rare central African animal or plant, being transferred to the monkeys by the bite of some insect—the funnel-webbed spider was suspect. The outbreak was quelled, but the disease could recur virulently anywhere in the world.

The lives the green monkeys took from man saved an infinite number of their own. They are now highly unpopular in civilization's laboratories.

# 21

## THE BLACK DEATH

### *A Clerical Disaster*

Shortly before the feast of St. John the Baptist in 1348, two ships from Bristol berthed at Melcombe in Dorset. One of the sailors had brought from Gascony "the seeds of the terrible pestilence." Melcombe enjoys remembrance as the first town in England ravaged by the Black Death.

*Pasteurella pestis* is a delicate round germ with a clear center. It is transmitted by rat fleas, producing bubonic plague with "buboes" of swollen lymph glands in the groin. The Black Death was its pneumonic form, a lethal infection causing gangrene of the lungs and passed around as easily as flu and colds.

The dead were black from hemorrhages into their skin. Corpses putrefied in houses and the streets, fearfully untouched. Pits were hastily dug and as rapidly filled—"the testator and his heirs and executors were hurled from the same cart into the same hole together." There was protection no more than from the lightning. Families burned juniper for fumigation, the sick tried blood-letting, or swallowing vinegar as advised by the "plague tracts." The physicians dressed up like modern surgeons, gloves, gown, mask with sponge soaked in cloves and cinnamon. Coast-dwellers put to sea and found the pestilence their cargo. Others fled their villages, forsaking friends, parents, children—efficiently spreading the infection.

The people had no doctors. They called in the clergy to save their lives by divine intercession, or failing that, their souls by confession. Over the winter of 1348, a hundred Dorset clergymen died. The vicars of Shaftesbury and Wareham were replaced four times between December and May. In neighboring Somerset, the usual nine new clergymen a month increased in December to 32, in January to 47, February to 43, March to 36. Forty-eight percent of the clergy died in the West Country diocese of Bath and Wells. The parishioners marveled at the man of God perishing just like his miserable sinners.

In January 1349, their bishop wrote:

> The contageous pestilence of the present day, which is spreading far and wide, has left many parish churches and other livings in our diocese without parson or priest to care for their parishioners. Since no priests can be found who are willing, whether out of zeal and devotion or in exchange for a stipend, to take on the pastoral care of these aforesaid places, nor to visit the sick and administer to them the Sacraments of the Church (perhaps for fear of infection and contagion), we understand that many people are dying without the Sacrament of Penance.

He announced a sensational emergency relaxation of canonical rules, permitting dying confession to another layman, "even to a woman." The bishop's exhortation dutifully to succor the sick was enfeebled by his passing the plague shut in his house in the inaccessible village of Wiveliscombe.

Of an English population of four million, 33 percent died in the Black Death. Of parish priests, 45 percent. Of the pious 17,500 secluded in monasteries and nunneries, 51 percent died from infection penetrating the susceptible cloisters.

Like the British army in World War I, the Church lost its best and keenest young officers. Like Britain afterward, it felt their lack. The sufferings of the Black Death left a land stirring with discontent and doubt, and left manor and parsonage ineffective to answer them. The dead clerics of 1348 were the first casualties of the Reformation of 1531.

It seems dreadfully unfair, or at least shortsighted, of God.

"How do you explain the scourges that afflict mankind?" a gentle old lady asked an abbé in *The Revolt of the Angels.* "Why are there plagues, famines, floods and earthquakes?"

"It is surely necessary that God should sometimes remind us of his existence," the abbé replied with a heavenly smile.

# 22

## THE RELUCTANT BENEFACTOR

### Stillbirth at St. Mary's

The discovery of penicillin *a disaster*? It is like complaining that the manna was not delivered from Heaven ready sliced.

The invisible penicillin mold did not descend equally miraculously upon Professor Alexander Fleming's poky laboratory in St. Mary's Hospital, London. It floated upstairs. The lab below was as thick with molds as a Neopolitan kitchen with flies. A man was spending his life studying them.

The mold fell upon the small glass plate of nutrient jelly coated with dangerous staphylococcus germs. (These would normally be developed in a laboratory incubator like a small oven, but Fleming had been examining the staphylococci for changes in color, more obvious if grown in the open air.)

It was August 1928. Fleming was off for a month's holiday in his native Scotland. He had finished his experiments, stacked his plates into a bucket of disinfectant. The top plate stood clear of the surface. The mold dropped on the germs at exactly the place and time to attack them. It was a dreadful summer, but the temperature that ruined Fleming's holiday was precisely right for nurturing his penicillin mold.

Back at work, Fleming noticed the forgotten top plate, with a murmur of "That's funny" examined it, discovered mold to be eating germs. (If you want to see for youself, the plate is in the British Museum.)

Fleming's discovery was the equivalent of an overjoyed bettor winning on six successive horses at the race track.

Taciturn, shy, academic Fleming saw penicillin mold as a laboratory tool, gobbling up ubiquitous staphylococci on plates of mixed germs—as from throat swabs—letting more interesting ones grow. Australian Howard Florey at Oxford created *the drug* penicillin in 1940. He came across Fleming's research, grew his own mold, refined it, and injected it into a patient at the Radcliffe Infirmary, all in 18 months. Florey had luck, too. His mind was conditioned by the later invention of germkillers. Germany had given the world the first sulpha drug, a month before bestowing upon it Hitler.

Florey made penicillin in milk bottles among the guinea pig hutches. The Americans made it in brewers' vats. As a minor disaster for Florey, the Americans also patented it and made the money.

There was enough penicillin for the wounded of Eisenhower's and Montgomery's armies by D-day. The disaster was Fleming missing its curative power in 1928. A mitigated one—penicillin was a weapon of war for the Allies, denied to the end the Nazis and Japanese.

# Part Five

# INSIDIOUS NATURE

# 23

## TRANSATLANTIC DISASTERS

### West and American Indian Revenge

November 24, 1494, brought the conjunction of Jupiter, Mars, and Saturn in the sign of the scorpion. This signaled an imminent outbreak of fearful venereal disease. The soothsayers spoke of little else.

On February 21, 1495, Charles VIII "The Affable" of France laid siege to Naples. (He did not *really* lay siege, he rode toward Vesuvius amid the tactful cheers of the populace.)

Naples was full of Spanish immigrants. In April 1493, Christopher Columbus had arrived in Barcelona from the Americas. A new disease shortly arrived in Barcelona. It caused spots all over, stinking ulcers, ravaging of the flesh, death, lingering agonies for the survivors. They had to build a special hospital in Seville. Nobody knew what to call it, until Hieronymus Frascastorious of Verona in 1530 hit on "Syphilis." That was the young shepherd who picked it up for annoying the gods. Columbus's sailors had picked it up in Haiti.

The Spaniards gave it to the Neapolitans, who called it the Spanish disease, who gave it to the French, who called it the Neapolitan disease and gave it to everybody. In the scurry to share the blame, the Poles called it the German disease and vice versa, the English (naturally) called it the French disease, and anyone short of foreign suspects could call it the Turkish disease, because the Turks had everything.

Explorers in Columbus's wake discovered the American Indians peacefully puffing their pipes. In 1565, the French Ambassador to Lisbon, Jean Nicot, presented an American tobacco plant to Queen Catherine de Medici, the king's mother, who ran France. He was honored by her christening it *Nicotina tabacum*.

Soon the pipes were lighting up all over Europe. Tobacco now causes 50,000 deaths a year in Britain, and with Voltairian irony 320,000 a year among the Europeans who sailed to spread themselves across the Redskins' fragrant forests, pure prairies, and refreshing rivers. A terrible ransom to extract for violation of privacy.

Thank God America today sends over nothing worse than Coca-Cola.

# 24

# CALAMITY IN THE CUPBOARD

## *Australian Disaster*

The equivalent for Australian palates of Thanksgiving turkey, the roast beef of Old England, *saltimbocca alla Romana,* Peking duck, Beluga caviar, *perdreau en crépine Brillat-Savarin*— possibly of all six combined—is the meat pie.

This is a small tank brimming with gravy the consistency of engine oil, the color of ashes, and the taste of sheepmeat boiled relentlessly and suspectedly whole. The filling has been compared in appearance to "what little babies do in their diapers." On biting the crust resembling soggy cardboard, the gravy escapes like superheated steam. To avoid a change of clothing, the pie must be sucked rather than chewed, in the position of bowing reverentially to the queen.

Such unexpected liquidity is insignificant to the thirsty inhabitants of a land two-thirds desert. They even soak the pie in ketchup. Some Australians emblazon all their food with ketchup—steak, eggs, French fries, oysters, asparagus, *pâté de foie gras.* One incredulous gourmet sampling Australia murmured, "Your kids take kitchup sauce sandwiches to school, and even have been known to put it on their ice cream."

Australians are addicted to sauces and in 1964, the poison of choice was Worcestershire sauce.

A 28-year-old housewife appeared in Brisbane Hospital with a stone in each kidney. Rigorous investigation on the couch, in the X-ray department, by the biochemistry laboratory, found no cause. Did she swallow popular pain-killers? asked the baffled doctors. These can create kidney stones. Overdose herself with vitamin D, in cranky health foods? Drink excessive milk? No? Well, was there *anything* unusual about her diet? Nothing at all, she replied. Unless you count Worcestershire sauce. She had a craving for it. She got through a bottle a day, even more when she was pregnant.

Worcestershire sauce! exclaimed the doctors. Full of acetic acid, which damages the kidney. Plus garlic, black pepper, ginger, allspice, mace, cinnamon, ingredients all containing volatile oils and equally nephrotoxic. She kicked the habit, the stones grew no bigger.

An earlier case then emerged, back in 1956, a bottle-a-day man.

Twelve months later, a 28-year-old painter appeared at the same hospital. He was a Scots immigrant, so well integrated in his new country he drank six pints of Foster's a day. He never touched milk.

He had two stones in his right kidney, seemingly without cause. Worcestershire sauce? asked the doctors. He was hooked on it. He swamped all his meals with it. His was an addiction tough to break. Like the wayward alcoholic anonymous, the first, quick dash from the bottle was the disastrous one. They dried him out saucewise and the stones stayed static.

I am a Worcestershire sauce buff. A Bloody Mary, a Welsh rarebit, an Irish stew, are as immemorable without it as a passionless kiss. After reading these cases, I gloomily struggled to renounce it, like cholesterol—a doctor, in the spirit of William Pitt's England, must save himself by his exertions and his patients by his example.

But this was *Australian* Worcestershire sauce. The distinction was made with dignified pique in the London *Times* by Mr. Lea, who with Mr. Perrins makes The Original and Genuine Worcestershire Sauce in Worcester (rhymes with Bertie Wooster), England. Each crimson label carries a brace of grouse, a hare, and their printed signature to discourage imitations, like the Bank of England's notes. The sauce contains shallots, tamarinds, and anchovies. It is made from the original recipe of a nobleman, perhaps the incandescent Sir Francis Dashwood of the Hell-fire Club.

No English nobleman would concoct anything remotely damaging to the kidney, an organ cherished by our aristocracy. How many armadas of champagne, port, claret, and burgundy have seeped through them since the Battle of Hastings! A peer in my London club—it still has gout-stools, to tuck to your chair and raise exquisitely painful toes to the easeful horizontal—so lingered in the bar that the ancient waiter respectfully reminded him of a grill long ordered. "My Lord, your kidneys are spoiling." "My God!" His lordship said, clasping his loins. "Is it beginning to show?"

I continue to sprinkle lavishly the English sauce so complimentary to English cooking, which is often inedible if you can taste it.

# 25

## ONE IN THE EYE

### *Celebratory Disaster*

Champagne!

"The only wine which leaves a woman beautiful after drinking it," said Madame de Pompadour. Declared Thackeray, "All enjoyments are sensual enjoyments. Shakespeare and Raphael never invented anything to equal champagne and oysters, at 5:30 on a hot day." Robert (Mr. Jorrocks) Surtees mixed it with apricot jam to clean his riding-boots. André Simon's habit of a bottle a day was broken only by death at 93. "My God, I am drinking stars!" exclaimed Dom Pérignon, who created it at Hautvillers Abbey near Epernay.

Dom Pérignon was the Faraday, the Watt, the Rutherford of enology. He invented the cork. He got the idea in the summer of 1694, when a pair of Spanish monks arrived with water flasks bunged by cork bark.

The pop of the champagne cork, as exuberant a consort of human joy as laughter itself, has a ghoulish echo of danger.

In swinging 1965, when Britons drank 5,181,185 bottles of champagne, eight Londoners between 24 and 72 years of age were taken to Moorfields Eye Hospital with injuries from the corks. Seven were serious enough for admission, three developed cataracts. Four of the eight patients were waiters. The relevant physics should be in the mind of anyone broaching a bottle of Cliquot.

Chilled champagne (47° F) has an intrabottle pressure of 90 pounds per square inch, rising at room temperature (65° F) and with shaking about. This can shoot the cork 40 feet. (A bottle of claret needs 300 pounds of force on the corkscrew to open it.) From the formula $V^2=U^2+2fs$ (V=initial U=final velocities in feet per second, f=acceleration of cork in feet per second, 2=distance in feet, while fiddling with the wire you can calculate that the cork strikes the eye with a velocity of 45 feet per second. It arrives in half the time of a blink, with a force of 100 atmospheres. This is comparable with blast injuries to the eye in mines and quarries.

To avoid ruining the party, champagne should be opened with a linen napkin over its mouth from the first breaking of the golden foil, the cork eased out pointing at someone else. The *Comité Interprofessional du Vin de Champagne* decrees white gloves, but this might be thought *outré* among the *canapés*. The "pop" is vulgar. There should be achieved the soft sibilance of an ecstatic sigh from a beautiful woman.

The injury would never have bothered Dom Pérignon himself. He was blind.

# 26

## SCURVY TREATMENT

### *Disastrous Diet for Gallant Gentlemen*

"The Great War, for instance, could never have happened if tinned food had not been invented," said George Orwell. All his insights were, of course, equally shrewd, but some more equally than others.

Without canned food, adventurous polar exploration certainly could never have happened.

On May 19, 1845, Captain Sir John Franklin, veteran of Copenhagen and Trafalgar at 19, sailed from Greenhithe in the Thames with HMS *Erebus* and *Terror* on his third Arctic expedition. The Admiralty had dispatched him to find the Northwest Passage. There would be a reward of £20,000.

Franklin provisioned for 137 men over 1,092 days. Each ship had a library of 1,200 books, volumes of *Punch,* and a barrel-organ that played 50 tunes, including ten hymns. His lavish stores included 33,289 pounds of preserved meat, Goldner Patent brand, in red tins.

Canning is as old as America. Frenchman Nicholas Appert in the eighteenth century preserved food by heat in sealed jars. Donkin and Hall of Blue Anchor Road in London's dockland were soon supplying the world with canned mutton and peas, boiled beef and carrots. (The roast veal of 1818 was enjoyed 120 years later by a venturesome English professor.) The Admiralty ordered canned meat aboard their ships as "medical comforts." Fresh-cooked meat would surely cure the scurvy.

Scurvy was a mysterious and terrible peril of the sea. The swollen, bloody, stinking gums, bruised skin, aching bones, and sudden death, were thought a contagion among men crammed into ships, camps, besieged cities. In the convict hulks off Woolwich it matched the hangman in efficiency. Or the cause was sea air, fit only for fish. Or it was punishment for laziness—lassitude being an early symptom.

A cure was found in 1597, scurvy-grass (a type of cress). God was well known to have given man diseases and a herb to cure each. But the concept of scurvy from *lack* of scurvy-grass was persistently beyond medical imagination, even into this century.

Sir Richard (South Seas) Hawkins cured scurvy in 1593 with oranges and lemons. Served years later, the East India Company issued lemon juice to all its ships. In 1773, naval surgeon James Lind of Edinburgh published *A Treatise of the Scurvy*, comparable in perception to William Harvey's treatise on the heart.

A year after Lind's death in 1794, and two hundred after Sir Richard Hawkins' idea, the Admiralty responded to Lind's urgings and provided lemon juice. The cases of scurvy in Haslar Naval Hospital dropped in ten years from 1,750 to one. Like Lister with hospital gangrene, Lind effected the cure without needing to know the cause.

Sir John Franklin sailed with 9,300 pounds of lemon juice in kegs, protected from freezing with a dash of rum. Each man took an ounce a day, diluted and sweetened, swallowed in the presence of an officer.

When Franklin had been away six-and-a-half years, people began to worry. After eight, further search was abandoned for an expedition provisioned only for three. On January 20, 1854, its officers and men were deemed to have died in Her Majesty's service.

Why, no one knew.

That October, Dr. John Rae of the Hudson Bay Company heard from Eskimos of 35 dead white men near the mouth of Great Fish River in King William Land, a hundred-mile long island well west of Baffin Land. Franklin's expedition had reached the eastern limits of the expeditions from the Pacific. He had succeeded. He had discovered the Northwest Passage existed.

Dr. Rae hastened to London with spoons, forks, and other relics of the lost men. The war had sucked British shipping to the Crimea. It was left for the Hudson Bay Company to organize a search party, which found seven hundred empty meat cans, arranged in regular rows. It seemed that Sir John Franklin had discovered his meat rotten, frantically ordered tin after tin broached, seen his expedition doomed by starvation. Britain erupted, particularly as the stuff was canned in Galatz, Moravia.

Lady Franklin bought a steam-yacht and mounted her own expedition. It discovered that *Erebus* and *Terror* had been trapped in the ice and abandoned on April 22, 1848, with 105 survivors reaching shore. Sir John had died on June 11, 1847, aged 61. Scurvy did for the rest.

The cooked meats and vegetables, were, in fact, fresh in their tins, but had no antiscorbutic vitamin C. This is destroyed by heat. The lemon juice, however, had after three years begun to decompose and was left aboard. The ships were plundered by the Eskimos and never seen again.

The Eskimos told of white men bleeding from the mouth, too weak to pull their sledges, struggling for the mainland of Canada. Vitamin C is synthesized by all animals except guinea-pigs and primates. Had the survivors caught fish and shot the Arctic deer and musk-cattle—not for nourishment but for their vitamins— they could have survived. U.S. Army Lieutenant Frederick Schwatka found their bones in 1878.

Sir John Franklin knew nothing about vitamins. Sir Frederick Gowland Hopkins of Cambridge won the Nobel Prize in 1929 for inventing them. In 1932, vitamin C was found chemically to be ascorbic acid. People now swallow it by the handful in the touching belief it keeps away colds.

# 27

## SANDWICH DISASTER

### Botulism on Loch Maree

Loch Maree is formed in Wester Ross, Scotland, by the river Garry. This rises on Ben Lair ten miles to the south, and continues northwest between flat, heather-speckled banks as the river Ewe, gathering large brooks which run down from the hill lochs. It flows into the Atlantic as Loch Ewe, opposite the north tip of Skye and the Outer Hebrides. It has fantastic sea-trout.

Loch Maree is fifteen miles by three, with half a dozen small islands in the middle, cradled by mountains reaching three thousand feet. The countryside is Nature's plain gift, barely refined by the artful hand of man; it has the simplicity the Scots so cherish in their scenery and their cooking.

On Monday, August 14, 1922, the bracken was starting to crisp but the evenings were still long, if chilly—frost was recorded that midnight at Glasgow. The day was overcast and sprinkled with showers. The forty-four guests who filled the famed Loch Maree Hotel enjoyed "a good, honest, wholesome, hungry breakfast" recommended by Izaak Walton, and split into fishing parties of two anglers per boat, with a ghillie to row. Fishermen intending to make a day of it were furnished with half a dozen sandwiches—cold meat, chicken-and-ham paste, and wild duck potted meat—prepared in the kitchen that morning.

The agreeable noonday moment arrived for unscrewing the

beer bottle, uncapping the hip flast, unwrapping the crinkly greaseproof paper. Major Anderson of the Seaforth Highlanders, on leave from India, preferred the cold beef. He passed the potted meat to his ghillie, though his wife Rosamund thought wild duck rather fun.

With the Great War barely four years dead, the holiday sparkled with rank. Brigadier-general Nichol found the potted duck nasty and lunched off cheese and biscuits. Colonel Lane finished his wild duck with relish. The gentlemen were so generous with sandwiches to the ghillies, young Ian Mackenzie could slip a selection into his creel for his wife.

The day's catch was weighed and laid in state on a marble slab in the hotel hall. The guests dressed and dined, to pass the evening with bridge and books. Before breakfast next morning, 22-year-old John Talbot, just down from Oxford, holidaying with his barrister father and his mother, complained of seeing double. As the news spread through the dining room, John Stewart—he was big in wool at Paisley—exclaimed that he, too, suffered the curious condition. He was puzzled at an inability to remove one of the two doughnuts on his plate. Everyone chortled. Seeing double? Been at the usquebaugh rather early in the day, old boy, eh what?

The two sufferers abandoned breakfast. They felt dizzy. Their eyelids began to droop. This was alarming. They felt tightening in the throat. They began to vomit and sweat. They staggered, had to lie down. Their speech became husky, indistinct, vanished. They could not swallow their spit. They could barely move arms and legs. They could hardly breathe. In his cottage along the Loch, ghillie Kenneth MacLennon was perplexed at his neighbor's smoking two pipes at once. Mrs. Rosamund Anderson and Mrs. Dixon, from Dublin, during the morning developed the same symptoms, by nightfall were dead. Mr. Talbot and Mr. Stewart died early next day. Brigadier-general Nichol and Colonel Lane felt fine.

The peaceful, pleasurable hotel held the horror of a country house mass-murder mystery. The remoteness that the holidaymakers had craved turned upon them terrifyingly. The nearest town was Gairloch, barely a thousand inhabitants, thirty miles from the railway, with no hospital nor telephone. The awesome double vision struck other trembling guests, the same symptoms ruthlessly followed, they went to their rooms and died.

Mrs. Dixon's husband died on Thursday morning, ghillie Mac-Lennon on Thursday night. On Monday, August 21, went 65-year-old Mr. Willis, another barrister from London (accompanied by his valet). Ghillie Mackenzie was the last, late Monday night, leaving a young widow and two children. "Happily, several medical men were staying in the hotel," *The Times* looked on the bright side, "and the sufferers had the best of care and attention."

Front-page headlines announced SCOTTISH POISON MYSTERY and DEADLY PASTE SANDWICHES. *The Times* carried black-edged columns, but because its owner, Lord Northcliffe, had died the same Monday (of syphilis, but nobody dared mention it).

The Loch Maree picnic captivated the public, like the equally inexplicable and chilling Loch Ness monster ten years later. The eight deaths were vaguely attributed to "ptomaine poisoning." Botulism was first mentioned on the Friday by the local Medical Officer of Health, Dr. Maclean, who had hurried cross-country from Dingwall by car.

Botulism is not the food poisoning that ruins Mediterranean and Mexican holidays. It is a sudden, violent, paralyzing nervous disease, caused by toxin from the germ *Clostridium botulinum*. The bacilli are short rods, which form resilient spores. They are scattered everywhere in the soil, useful in the decomposition of dead animals and plants. They grow only *without* oxygen—as in a jar of potted meat heated insufficiently, in the factory, to kill the spores. (Sausages in Latin are *botuli*.)

Botulinus toxin has the dangerous idiosyncracy of acting when swallowed. To get tetanus from its brother *Clostridium tetani*, you have to cut yourself. Antitoxin treatment is unlikely to save life once symptoms appear. If you suffer double vision after potted meat, do not take a taxi to the hospital, scream for an ambulance.

Loch Maree was the first outbreak of botulism in Britain. A previous outbreak in Europe was twenty-five years earlier, three Germans dying after eating ham. One in America was only two months before, six dead in Idaho from home-canned vegetables. In the United States, home canning was more dangerous than home brewing. (Only fruit is safe, the acidity kills the bacillus).

An inquiry under Scotland's Sudden Deaths Act convened a fortnight later at Dingwall, with Sheriff Mackintosh sitting and a jury. It emerged that the wild duck paste was bought from an Inverness grocer in June, a consignment of two dozen glass jars from Lazenby's of London (Est. 1795). Lazenby's had been potting duck in their Bermondsey factory for 35 years, 700 jars to the batch. They bought the wild duck in Leadenhall Poultry Market, just like the Savoy Hotel. Only one pot of the paste was infected.

Lazenby's dispatched north a King's Counsel with a watching brief. Dr. Maclean revealed that he had just consumed, in the cause of truth and science, a tin of Maconachie's rations intended for the Boer War. Counsel asked, "You suffered no ill effects?" "Well, I am still here." (*Laughter.*) It was a tragedy too baffling to take seriously.

Like the magistrate contemplating the death of young Albert Ramsbottom, eaten by the lion at Blackpool in Stanley ("Alfred Doolittle") Holloway's monologue, Sheriff Mackintosh comfortably "gave his opinion that no one was really to blame." If the jury was a generation ahead of its time in demanding "sell-by" dates on groceries, four of its seven were women.

The deadly jar must somehow have escaped sterilization in Bermondsey. It was a disaster for the canned food trade for years. Lloyd's of London offered hotels and boardinghouses insurance against food poisoning, £1,000 cover for half-a-crown a bed. A can of Alaskan salmon as a treat for tea was as lethal 56 years later in the British midlands. It cost the canners two million pounds. In 1982, a Belgian died from salmon canned at Ketchycan, Alaska. A puncture in a few cans, hidden by the label, necessitated the recall of five million others. The same year, botulism struck the Thames, ravaging the swans. Luckily, it turned out the wrong diagnosis. It was lead poisoning from the anglers' weights.

Loch Maree was the only instance in history of Russian roulette played with sandwiches.

# Part Six

# RIGHT IS WRONG

# 28

## DOCTOR DEATH

### *Nemesis on the Dawn Express*

George Orwell dates the decline of the English murder from 1925, when the perfect crime for the Sunday papers was perpetuated by "A little man of the professional class—a dentist or a solicitor, say—living an intensely respectable life somewhere in the suburbs, and preferably in a semi-detached house, which will allow the neighbors to hear suspicious sounds through the wall. . . . He should plan it all with the utmost cunning, and only slip up over some tiny unforseeable detail."

Murderers, like garage mechanics, have lost love for their work. They shoot, knife, bludgeon, and flee, instead of plotting with devilish ingenuity. Such carelessness does not mirror their relief from errors costing their life. Exceptional cleverness, infinite pains, fail hopelessly to outwit the modern police laboratory.

The salutarily inhibiting science of forensic medicine was invented by Sir Bernard Spilsbury, of Oxford and St. Mary's Hospital, London.

In 1910, Spilsbury examined "the remains," dug from Dr. Crippen's suburban cellar, identified them as Mrs. Cora Crippen despite lack of limbs, bones, genital organs, and head (none ever found), and discovered them full of poisonous hyoscine. The tabloid readers of the world relished the torments of the down-at-heel doctor from Coldwater, Michigan, fleeing home across the

Atlantic with his typist, Ethel le Neve, disguised as a boy, "trapped by wireless," overtaken by a Scotland Yard inspector in a fast liner, arrested on the St. Lawrence river, brought back in handcuffs, and tried in pomp at the Old Bailey. Thirty-three-year-old Spilsbury was like an unknown tenor making his name in a gala performance at Covent Garden.

He appeared with all the greats of murder in its greatest age.

In 1912, he was seen opposite Frederick Seddon, the London insurance agent who gave arsenic from flypapers to his lady lodger for her £4,000 life's savings. In 1915 with Brides in the Bath specialist George Smith, who did for three of them under the taps. In 1922 with Herbert Armstrong, the churchwarden who poisoned his wife and was charged in the remote Welsh court where he sat as clerk—which had no lamps and needed to adjourn when daylight faded.

During 1924, Patrick Mahon cut Emily Kay into little bits, boiling some of her in a saucepan on the living room fire, grinding the bones, and scattering her all over his seaside bungalow at the Crumbles, near Beachy Head. Spilsbury caught the Eastbourne express from Victoria, fitted her together like a three-dimensional jigsaw, even found her two months pregnant. For the first time he gave the full service, including postmortem after execution.

Spilsbury shared the limelight with butcher Louis Voison, who put his mistress's torso in a sack labelled *Argentina La Plata Cold Storage* during a Zeppelin raid. Then appeared with the famous duo Edith Thompson and Frederick Bywaters, a seafarer with the stylish P. & O. line, both hanged for knifing her husband in the East London suburb of Ilford (Spilsbury thought Edith was guiltless).

It was fashionable among murderers before World War Two to dismember their victims, pack them in trunks, and leave them at railway stations. Mr. Crossman cemented Mrs. Crossman into a tin trunk in 1902. Mr. Devereux dispatched his wife and twin children in similar luggage to a furniture depository in 1905. Nineteen twenty-seven brought the Charing Cross Station trunk murder (wickerwork trunk covered with black oilcloth), 1933 the first Brighton one (plywood covered with brown canvas, legs in a suitcase at King's Cross), a month later the second Brighton one (black canvas). In 1935 no trunk, but legs and feet with corns under a carriage seat at Waterloo.

Spilsbury's hands were in all this baggage. The coincidence of trunks and torsos fascinates the public like beds and actresses. He rocketed to the popularity of Sherlock Holmes. (Murderers have gone off trunks. This is from the international decrepitude of railways, and the fad for compact baggage necessitating a hard night's work with the food processor.)

Spilsbury manipulated scalpel, microscope, and test-tube with dour thoroughness. To find the effect of a bullet through skin, he cadged an amputated leg from a surgeon and peppered it with a revolver. To test his theory on the brides in the bath, he had a St. Mary's nurse volunteer for a tub (scientific accuracy assumedly precluding a swimsuit), ducking her with an unexpected tug of the legs. "The nurse in question nearly died," the director of public prosecutions revealed later.

No case was buried with its victim. Spilsbury took the first train and dug it up.

> When arsenic has closed your eyes,
> This certain hope your corpse may rest in:
> Sir B. will kindly analyse
> The contents of your large intestine.

said *Punch* beneath his cartoon in rubber gloves and apron, wing collar and lavender spats.

He was tall and handsome, dressed by Savile Row, bowler-hatted by Lock of St. James's, red carnation always in buttonhole. His shirt sleeves detached at the elbow, to save creasing the cuffs from repeated rolling-up. All doctors develop a bedside manner, Spilsbury a dockside one. In the witness box he combined the assurance of God with the menace of the Devil. He was brief, clear, decisive, as untechnical as the medical columns of the picture papers. Juries loved him because they could understand him. Judges the more so, because they needed not take the trouble to. He was ruffled only once, when insinuating his overwhelming medical authority to a junior barrister who responded, "When did you last examine a *live* patient, Sir Bernard?"

A murder trial without Spilsbury was as unthinkable as *Cinderella* without the Fairy Godmother. His opinions were so impregnable he could achieve single-handed all the legal consequences of homicide—arrest, prosecution, conviction, and final postmortem—requiring only the brief assistance of the hangman.

This reputation was perhaps as deterrent as the rope itself. A killer might think twice, aware that the next morning Spilsbury would be sitting in a first-class carriage from London.

But was it possible that Spilsbury and his reputation were as threatening to the innocent as to the guilty?

Three months after Patrick Mahon was hanged for the Crumbles crime, Elsie Cameron was murdered by young Norman Thorne on a poultry farm twenty miles away across Sussex. He sawed her into four portions, crammed her head in a cookie-tin, wrapped the rest in sacking, and buried her under his Leghorns. When questioned, he explained that she had arrived at his bungalow threatening to stay until he married her. He went out to the movies and came home to find her hanging from a beam. He cut her up in panic. So said Crippen about his Cora.

The police dug Elsie up for Spilsbury, 43 days after death. The trial, in the spring of 1926, occurred, like Mahon's, in the beautiful County Hall of Lewes. The wigs, the robes, the golden Royal Arms, the beautifully polished oak, the decorative judge, dignified counsel, and decorous bobbies, afford an out-of-town murder trial the cosy charm of an English tea party, with the incidental excitement that the guest of honor might be handed a poisoned cucumber sandwich.

Thorne's neck depended upon some marks on Elsie's. Spilsbury could find no signs of hanging, only the normal skin creases. He thought she had been hit on the head and strung up.

For the defense was pathologist Robert Brontë, a talkative Irishman. He found the mark of a thin rope. So did six other doctors. Spilsbury countered that Brontë had examined the body 47 days after he did, for 28 of which it was buried in the London suburb of Willesden, so not in prime condition. "I have had over twenty years continuous experience of microscopic work and the making of slides, applied more especially to medical-legal problems," he crushed the court.

Elsie Cameron was a neurotic. Even balanced young people impulsively kill themselves from frustrated passion. Though it was seven to one against, the jury decided Dr. Brontë's evidence as imaginative as *Wuthering Heights*.

The prisoner was condemned, the press indicted Spilsbury. "The unquestioning acceptance by the jury of Sir Bernard Spilsbury's evidence . . . the singling out of this particular medical witness for eulogy by the judge, seems a legitimate point for comment." The *Law Journal* objected that the court "followed the man with the biggest name." Conan Doyle was outraged. Perhaps he perceived, like Whistler, that Nature was creeping up on his art.

Toward midnight on October 23, 1929, there was a fire at the Metropole Hotel Margate—a bleak and tawdry resort on the Kent coast—in which 63-year-old Mrs. Rosaline Fox was suffocated in her undershirt. She was staying there with her 30-year-old son Sidney, in the room next door. On November 9, Spilsbury was on the express from Liverpool Street Station to Norwich. Mrs. Fox was born in the Norfolk village of Great Frensham, where she had been buried for ten days.

The coffin was sealed with putty, the body beautifully fresh. Spilsbury found a bruise behind the larynx. A Margate doctor said she died from shock and suffocation, the Margate coroner that hers was death by misadventure. Spilsbury said it was by strangulation. Sidney Fox was charged with murder. The case was transferred from Kent to the same lovely courtroom in Lewes where Spilsbury and Brontë again confronted each other.

Brontë had seen no bruise. Spilsbury objected that Brontë got his hands on the body when putrefication made the bruise unrecognizable. Brontë responded that Spilsbury could not tell bruising from putrefication. Fox was hanged.

That Fox was a swindler, a bilker of hotel bills, a flaunting homosexual, had been jailed for theft and forgery, had £3,000 worth of insurance policies on his mother's life, all expiring that same midnight, was beside the point. He was hanged because a jury believed a bruise was there, simply because Spilsbury said so.

Like Noël Coward and the Duke of Windsor, Spilsbury did not fit comfortably into the world left by Hitler's war. At the Tottenham Court Road murder of April 1947, he was far from himself. His doctor son had been killed in an air raid, another died of TB. He suffered three strokes and from arthritis. On December 17 he performed a postmortem in Hampstead, dined at his club, and gassed himself in his laboratory in University College, Bloomsbury.

Spilsbury did 25,000 postmortems. About 250 of his subjects were murdered. If his evidence was wrong with only 3.3 percent of them, his victims equalled Jack the Ripper's eight.

# 29

# IRONING OUT THE BUGS IN PANAMA

## *Colonel Gorgas vs. the U.S. Army*

It was not stout Cortez with a wild surmise about a Panama canal. It was his cousin Alvaro de Saavedra Ceron. It was not even Cortez on September 25, 1513, who stared silent upon a peak in Darien. It was Balboa, who would have ruined the scansion.

The German Emperor Charles V—he had inherited Spain from his mother—thought a canal at Panama the greatest idea since the chastity-belt. But frustrated by politics and tormented by gout, Charles abdicated in 1555 to live his last three years in a monastery. His son, Philip II, declared the canal impious. Those oceans whom God hath set asunder let no man join together. He decreed death even for thinking of it.

William Paterson, the Scotsman who founded the Bank of England, in 1698 floated the "Darien Scheme" from the Bahamas. The Spanish-owned isthmus would enjoy the infinite benefit of a Scottish colony, becoming a tradesman's entrance to the Pacific, "Whereby to Britain would be secured the key to the universe, enabling their possessors to give laws to both oceans and to become arbiters of a commercial world."

On July 26 the Scots sailed from Leith, christened their wedge of the Isthmus New Caledonia, its unbuilt cities New Edinburgh and New St. Andrews. Within a year, starvation, sickness, and the Spaniards saw them off. The investors lost all their money (as have many since, with financial schemes conceived in the Bahamas).

Twenty-one-year-old Horatio Nelson first saw active service in 1780, sailing a frigate to San Juan, 250 miles north of Panama in Nicaragua. The expedition was a disaster. Of his crew of 200, 190 died of fever, and Nelson himself fell sick and was nearly lost to glory.

The trans-Isthmus railway was built in 1855 by Americans William E. Howland and William H. Aspinwall, with the help of Chinese and Irish laborers who died with the near predictability of hogs herded into Chicago slaughterhouses.

In 1876 man and geography were ready to be matched in mortal combat.

The Suez Canal had been opened on November 17, 1869, by the Empress Eugénie sailing in the French imperial yacht *Aigle*. Her cousin Ferdinand de Lesseps had become the world's greatest hero since Alexander the Great and its most famous benefactor since the Good Samaritan. If a Frenchman could pierce Suez and Mont Cenis, why should a few sandbanks and lumps of rock frustrate his ravishment of Panama?

In 1876 the *Société Civile Internationale du Canal Interocéanique* was formed in Paris. In May 1878 it sent Lieutenant L. N. Bonarparte-Wyse to reconnoiter. He brought home the canal concession from the Colombian government. The *Société* sold it to de Lesseps' Panama Canal Company for 10 million francs. On New Year's Day 1880, de Lesseps' little granddaughter administered the first *coup de pioche,* and there was a gala performance at the Panama theater with Sarah Bernhardt. De Lesseps was 74.

Extravagance, corruption, dishonesty, and greed were the canal-diggers' unseen enemies. The Colombia courts multiplied land values a thousand times, the French as eagerly paid up. The *Aëdes aegypti* mosquito was their barely visible deadly one. It bore on its wings yellow fever.

The death rate among de Lesseps's men settled down at 176 per thousand. Of 86,800 employees over eight years, 52,814 fell ill and 5,627 died. The French found no cold season to kill off the germs. Only the wet season from April to December when you were liable to die in three days from yellow fever, and the dry season from December to April when you were liable to die in 24 hours from pernicious fever.

There were 624 deaths in October 1884. Monkey Hill outside Colon became congested with forty funerals a day. A shipment of 500 young French engineers all died in the swamps before they could draw their first month's pay. In September 1884 the entire crew died of yellow fever aboard a British brig anchored off Colon. The French allowed only 0.5 percent of their budget for hospitals, for sanitation nothing at all. In 1888 the Panama Canal Company went bankrupt.

Nothing is more dangerous than the buckled lance of *amour-propre*. Furious France indicted Ferdinand de Lesseps and his son Charles with breach of trust. (The government anyway needed scapegoats to protect the Third Republic from its gleeful enemies.) Father and son got five years. Ferdinand was too ill to imprison, he died poor and embittered at La Chenaie on December 7, 1894, a victim of yellow fever, second-hand.

Anthony Froude wrote at the time, "In all the world there is not perhaps now concentrated in any single spot so much swindling and villainy, so much foul disease, such a hideous dung-heap of physical and moral abomination. The Isthmus is a damp, tropical jungle, intensely hot, swarming with mosquitoes, snakes, alligators, scorpions, and centipedes; the home, even as Nature made it, of yellow fever, typhus and dysentery."

The 40-mile-wide Isthmus was a tangle of vegetation, palms, mangroves, and creepers, alive with monkeys, parrots, vividly plumaged birds, wild turkeys, wild boar and hogs, snakes, lizards, and tarantulas. The flowers, though, were lovely. The orchids, in particular, had tempted several zealous botanists to their graves. There was frequent lightning, more frequent rain. It was a dank terror abuzz with mosquitoes. Just the challenge for Americans to prove themselves better men than the French.

America needed a Panama Canal to safeguard her national interest as the British needed the Straits of Dover. In February 1904 the Senate ratified a canal treaty with the three-month-old Republic of Panama. It would be dug by the U.S. Army Corps of Engineers, under an Isthmian Canal Commission headed by Colonel G. W. Goethals. It would cost $156,378,258.

The Americans arrived to find disintegrating French machinery, rusting locomotives growing trees, buildings half-digested by the jungle. Perhaps they felt the familiarity with death of Walter Scott's Sergeant More McAlpin, whose habitual morning walk was beneath the elms of the churchyard. New York could proudly call itself "The Empire State." Panama had won the title of "The White Man's Grave."

In June 1904 Colonel William Crawford Gorgas of the U.S. Army Medical Corps arrived with five other doctors and Miss Hibberd, a nurse. Colonel Gorgas had lived with yellow fever as comfortably as Sherlock Holmes with crime.

Yellow fever is ferocious jaundice. A fulminating, massive infection of the liver, the body's powerhouse. It starts with rocketing fever, up to 106 degrees Farenheit, with backache, headache, photophobia, and prostration. Next, bleeding from the mouth, nose and gums, bleeding into the skin, bleeding unseen into the gut. Then the jaundice and vomiting, ending with the notorious "black vomit" of broken-down blood exuded into the stomach.

The kidneys and the bone-marrow go the way of the liver, the patient stops passing urine and making blood cells, turns delirious, slips from convulsions to coma, dies. Yellow fever lurks still in tropical Africa and central and south America, the traveler safeguarded by immunization with the attenuated living vaccine. The germ is an RNA arbovirus (ribonucleic acid arthropodborne), its reservoir monkeys. The incubation period is three to six days.

Gorgas was born in 1854 at Mobile, under the stimulating prenatal influence of Dr. Josiah Nott, the first doctor to suggest that mosquitoes might spread yellow fever. "Yellow Jack" was also "Yellow Breeze," believed to be borne by the wind. Or by oranges and bananas, frenziedly burnt by the crateful during epidemics.

Gorgas was medicine's action man. He first wanted to kill people, and tried joining the army. Throwing his energies into reverse, he graduated from Bellevue Hospital, New York, in 1880. *Then* he joined the army. His enthusiasm was directed to yellow fever, which had weighed heavily on the military mind since it killed more Americans from 1846 to 1848 than had the Mexicans.

Gorgas was posted to Fort Brown, Texas, and placed under arrest for entering the off-limits fever ward.

His colonel's daughter, Miss Doughty Lyster, caught yellow fever. Her own doctor evaluated her chances of recovery by ordering her grave to be dug. Colonel Lyster woefully invited Gorgas— as a professional man, in the lack of a chaplain—to conduct the funeral service. Gorgas briskly agreed, but was forestalled by both the patient getting better and catching yellow fever himself. His attack was slight. He convalesced with Doughty, fell in love, and married her, his happiness complete by now being immune to yellow fever for life.

In 1898 Gorgas cleaned up Havana. He believed like everyone else that yellow fever was caused by "filth," and started vigorously making the place "as cleanly as Fifth Avenue." His passion was disastrously misplaced. The yellow fever got worse. Not among the poor Cubans in their insanitary hovels (they were immune). Among the 25,000 settlers from Spain and the United States in their airy spotless dwellings (they were not). Cleanliness seemed as desirable as innocence amid thieves.

The military governor died of yellow fever. So did the chief commissary of the army. His widow *wanted* to die of yellow fever, and attempted suttee by rolling in the black vomit which plastered her husband's corpse. It did not work, so she shot herself. The commanding general's staff officer attended her funeral, caught yellow fever, and died in four days. It was a dreadful week.

The origin of yellow fever was as baffling as the origin of the universe. You did not catch it from someone, like a cold. How otherwise would the commissary's widow have survived that poisonous vomit? She had no earlier attack and no immunity. (As Queen Victoria had luckily won immunity to typhoid, before she frantically kissed her husband's typhoid-slain corpse at Windsor Castle in 1861.)

There was Dr. Henry Carter's mysterious "period of extrinsic incubation." You got yellow fever from visiting a friend who was recovering after a fortnight, but never if you compassionately hastened around as soon as he fell sick. There was the ghostly "Bacillus X," until Surgeon-General Sternberg exorcised it in 1900. Then Dr. Carlos Finlay revived the idea of mosquitoes.

Dr. Finlay was a friend of Gorgas, amiably sceptical of his

Operation Fifth Avenue in Havana. Major Walter Reed of Virginia had just arrived there. He thought mosquitoes, too. He had the satisfaction of producing fourteen cases among his friends, by submitting them to mosquito bites or injections of patients' blood. He had seven enlisted men sleep in beds just vacated by yellow fever victims. None got it. His colleague, Dr. Jesse W. Lazear made a sad final sentence to the chapter of yellow fever disasters, by dying after an accidental mosquito bite.

The *Aëdes aegypti* mosquito stood indicted and convicted of mass murder. Its criminal *modus operandi* was sucking blood in the first three days of fever, developing the disease in its body, and passing it on after twelve. Young mosquitoes that fed by day were seldom infected. The old ones fed at evening and early morning, danger times. A mosquito once infected stayed infective for life. Gorgas threw mosquito-proof screens around his patients and instantly mounted a powerful search-and-destroy operation against mosquitoes. He freed Havana from yellow fever for the first time in 150 years. Then he traveled to the end of the Great American Rainbow in Panama.

Gorgas did not officially exist. He had neither government funds, backing, nor encouragement. His sanitary regulations were either rejected or unenthusiastically imposed and ignored by the workers. Admiral J. G. Walker of the Canal Commission knew his own mind. "I am not going to spend good American dollars on a group of insane enthusiasts who spend their time chasing mosquitoes. Chasing mosquitoes through the Panama jungle seems to me the very height of folly. Even the French in their wildest moments never did anything as bad as that. As everyone knows, what causes yellow fever is not mosquitoes but filth and dirt."

"Sanitation!" cried General G. W. Davis, first governor of the Canal Zone. "What has that to do with digging the canal? Spending a dollar on sanitation is as good as throwing it into the bay. It's for your own good, Gorgas, I say this," he advised benevolently. "You have harped on the mosquito idea until it has become an obsession, and your assistants have caught it, too. Oh do, for goodness sake get it out of your head! Yellow fever, as we all know, is caused by filth."

Colonel Goethals himself was more analytical. "Do you know,

Gorgas, that every mosquito you kill costs the U.S. government ten dollars?"

"But just think, Colonel Goethals," Gorgas replied pleasantly. "One of those ten dollar mosquitoes might bite you, and what a loss that would be to the country."

A hideous, swiftly fatal disease borne by gossamer-winged mosquitoes! As ridiculous to men who thought of death in terms of batteries and battleships as the suggestion of man-eating butterflies. The French failed at Panama through mismanagement and waste. The Americans would win through stringent economy. These robust sentiments were all uttered in Washington, D.C. The Commission saw no reason for visiting Panama. They might catch yellow fever.

There was no yellow fever when Gorgas arrived at Panama in June 1904. The disease had left with the French. There were no susceptible strangers to catch it. December saw 6 cases and one death.

January 1905, 19 cases and 8 deaths. On New Year's Eve, officers of the U.S. cruiser *Boston* in Colon harbor had thrown a party. One mild case of yellow fever was unknowingly invited, a fortnight later six of the crew went down. April brought 9 cases and 2 deaths. May, 33 cases, 8 deaths. In June there were 62 cases and 19 deaths. In July there was panic.

An epidemic! Everyone wanted to go home. Engineers, clerks, cooks, laborers, shopkeepers. The canal could be abandoned. The greatest American dream since Independence itself was vanishing through the everyday disaster of not doing what your doctor told you.

But they could not go home. The only escape from Panama was by water, as from Alcatraz. There were no ships. By the time a rescue flotilla was mustered they might be all dead. They could only stare at each other with a wild surmise they might be developing yellow fever. They began to consider that there might be something in those goddam mosquitoes after all.

Gorgas swung into action.

If you wanted water in Panama, you had to wait until it rained. It was collected and stored near the houses in an infinite variety of domestic utensils. The mosquitoes laid eggs on the water—the outbreak aboard the *Boston* came from a *purée* of mosquito larvae in a pan outside the galley. Gorgas's restive memory recalled fever vanished from New York when the water vanished into pipes. Eliminate standing water, eliminate yellow fever.

Colonel Gorgas divided his forces. The *Aëdes* Brigade would attack the mosquitoes of yellow fever. The *Anopheles* Brigade those of malaria. He established the criminal offense of harboring mosquito larvae, fine five dollars. A mosquito needs little room for reproduction. Crevices in stones, thrown out cans, holy water stoups in churches, all made love nests. An outbreak in the hospital was traced to the little dishes of water under the legs of the food safe to keep out the ants.

Gorgas advanced on the vegetation with flame throwers. The captured enemy was chloroformed and microscoped, to determine its precise regiment in the swarming army. All patients were camouflaged with mosquito netting. A phone call to the Sanitary Squad, reporting marauding mosquitoes, instantly produced a truck with a sanitary inspector and half a dozen men, crawling all over your house with flashlights. You would not get that sort of service today, even reporting a cellarful of dead rats.

In a brilliant strategic stroke, Gorgas deployed large, flat, scoured pans of fresh water, so inviting that the *Aëdes aegypti* mosquitoes hastened to lay their eggs—then Gorgas outwitted the foe by tipping the lot down a disinfected drain. The yellow fever mosquito fancied clean water and bred close to houses. The malaria mosquito bred anywhere. Gorgas vigorously drained the swamps. There was hardly a puddle left. Panama had 8 million feet of ditches, and every stream painstakingly polluted with a film of oil.

In September 1906, Gorgas—no firefly under a bushel— boasted, "In six months I have rid the Isthmus of yellow fever— after four hundred years!" Then Secretary of War Taft fired him.

During 1906, the American Medical Association had sent a Dr. Charles Reed snooping around Panama. The AMA entertained doubts about the collaboration of the Isthmian Commission with its medical staff.

Dr. Reed discovered that if, say, the superintendent of Ancon Hospital in Panama needed supplies, he sent the appropriate form to the chief sanitary officer, who sent it to the governor of the Zone, who sent it to the chief disbursing officer, who sent it to the

Isthmian Canal Commission, who sent it to a member of the Commission detailed to specialize in such things, who sent it back to the Isthmian Canal Commission, who, if they approved of it, invited bids from contractors by sending it to their purchasing agent (who was not expected to know anything about sanitation), who sent the article to the Isthmus care of the chief of the Bureau of Materials and Supplies, who—the pace now hots up—sent it to the chief disbursing officer who had first mailed the form to the Commission, who passed the consignment to Colonel Gorgas, who presented it to the hospital superintendent, if he was lucky. Up-and-coming America in Panama was determined to muddle through as steadfastly as complacent Britain in the Crimea. Gorgas and the vigorous Miss Nightingale would have made a lovely couple.

Teddy Roosevelt got to hear about this and changed the system. He also made all Commission members go and live in Panama. The President had earlier appointed Governor Shonts there. Shonts wanted to replace Gorgas with a friend of his own in the medical line, an osteopath. Quite right, agreed Mr. Secretary Taft, who concurred with Governor Shonts that the cause of yellow fever was bad smells. Taft had sniffed for himself, and Panama smelt as bad as ever. All Gorgas did in Panama was to endanger the success of the entire scheme.

This could have been the most disastrous disaster of all. Gorgas went, but luckily his work remained. The death rate in the Canal Zone by 1914 was 6.2 per thousand, compared with that of the entire United States, 14.1 per thousand.

William Gorgas died on July 3, 1920, at Queen Alexandra's Military Hospital, Millbank, London. He was visiting the capital of so much potentially pestiferous land that the sun never set on it.

King George V had made him a knight (honorary). The British gave him St. Paul's for his funeral. His country buried him in Arlington. Gorgas has been meanly criticized as a scientist who never discovered, but won his reputation from the discoveries of others. But as his contemporary, Sir William Osler of Oxford remarked: "In science, the credit goes to the man who convinces the world, not the man to whom the idea first occurs."

On Thursday, November 20, 1913, the first ship sailed through the canal. She was the French *Louise,* which 25 years before had taken de Lesseps back to France. Brash America was determined to make a *beau geste* as handsomely as polished France.

The finished canal followed the same route as suggested by Alvaro de Saavedra Ceron in 1523.

# 30

## Untreasured Island

### *How to Beat Hitler with Sheep*

"We shall fight on the beaches," Winston Churchill challenged during the disastrous Dunkirk week of June 1940. "We shall fight on the landing grounds, we shall fight in the fields and in the streets, we shall fight in the hills."

He might have added, "And on a small island off the northwest coast of Scotland, with rather more chance of success."

Hitler and his friends were in charge from Tokyo Bay to Algeciras Bay, from Murmansk to Mersa Matrûh. There was nothing that lovely summer to stop him shooting the bluebirds and landing on the White Cliffs of Dover.

The British, with customary endearing crankiness, set about defending their precious stone set in a silver sea. All signposts were removed, so Nazi parachutists, invariably dressed as nuns, would betray themselves at rustic crossroads with paroxysms of Teutonic choler over the correct route from Husbands Bosworth to Husborne Crawley, or if in Wales from Llansantffraid Glyn-Ceirog to Llansantffaid yn Mechain.

The fields were scattered with oil drums, spiky harrows, rusty potato-planters and broken-down tractors, scarecrows against more Nazi nuns arriving by glider. The shore was unwelcoming with prickly lengths of railway track. British housewives beat their aluminum saucepans into Spitfires. Nothing was too devil-ish for Hitler.

Dr. Paul Fildes, of the Chemical Defense Experimental Estab-lishment, gazed through his laboratory window across the lovely Wiltshire countryside of Porton Down and dreamed of anthrax.

The *Bacillus anthracis* is a microbial giant, a square-ended rod generally going about in pairs. On nutrient jelly it grows grayish, feltlike blobs, with tangled edges microscopically resembling curly hair—the "Medusa head." One glance from Gorgon Me-dusa instantly turned you to stone, one touch from the anthrax bacillus could be equally calamitous.

There are two sorts of anthrax. One from an infected scratch, a black scab surrounded by bursting blebs of skin, with the trivial mortality of 25 percent. And anthrax of the lungs, "woolsorters' disease," described in a 1940 textbook of medicine with gusto: "Onset rapid. Rigor, rapid respiration, pain in chest, rapid and feeble pulse. Cough and bronchitis usual. *Temperature high.* Edema of chest wall develops, of gelatinous consistency. Much frothy mucus. Extreme collapse and death in one to three days."

Exactly what any Englishman would then have wished any German, particularly as the account ends, "Mind usually re-mains clear."

Anthrax was a disease of farmers and vets and men working in slaughterhouses. No one had thought of it as a weapon of war before. The difficulty was extending these startling effects to the entire population of the Ruhr. Dr. Fildes knew you sometimes got it from shaving brushes, but this did not seem enormously useful, apart from humanely sparing the women and children.

It was no problem in a summer of desperate resourcefulness, when old ladies learned to mix (later named) Molotov cocktails, and when the rifleless Home Guard commandeered pitchforks to stick into the descending buttocks of parachuting nuns. The RAF diverted briefly from the Battle of Britain to design anthrax bomblets.

These bomblets would be packed with billions of anthrax spores, disseminated with a small, economical charge. A recom-mendation for bombarding the Germans with anthrax rather than, say, *Pasteurella pestis* of the Black Death, was this handy ability of each microbe to armor itself with a thick spore. Once again in a warm, moist, airy environment with its customary nutrients, the spore became its old self and ready to fight for king and country.

The next task was trying out the secret weapon. The army's traditional testing ground of Salisbury Plain carried the disadvantage of possibly wiping out the inhabitants of Salisbury. So many unlikely corners of the British Isles were already commandeered for military use—divers jostled with the Monster in Loch Ness, St. James's Park opposite Buckingham Palace was full of antiaircraft balloons, Brighton front was thick with pillboxes camouflaged as ice cream kiosks.

The War Office swooped on Gruinard Island. It was a mile long and half a mile wide. It stood a couple of miles offshore in hilly Gruinard Bay, which looked northeast from the convoluted Wester Ross coast across the North Minch toward Stornoway in the Outer Hebrides. Better still, it was uninhabited.

In the spring of 1941, when London, Coventry, and elsewhere had been ravaged by the Luftwaffe, when Roosevelt had pushed Lend Lease through Congress, when Hitler was contemplating invading Russia, and when his Deputy-Führer was contemplating dropping into the Duke of Hamilton from his Messerschmitt 150 miles to the south, Dr. Fildes was ready at Gruinard Island.

He arrived with several army trucks full of sheep. Sixty hapless baaing contributors to the war effort were ferried across the bay, tethered to stakes scattered over the rock-strewn Gruinard grass beneath gantries of poles and planks, and showered with anthrax spores from exploded bomblets. The experiment was successful beyond its engineer's dreams. Every sheep was shortly dead.

The rest was pencil-and-paper work.

Anthrax was clearly more effective than TNT. The British, before the Blitz, awarded each ton of Nazi bombs a "multiplier" of 50, meaning fifty civilian casualties. (This was flattering the Luftwaffe, which in the Spanish Civil War achieved a multiplier of only 17.2.) The inhabitants of Berlin, Frankfurt, Stuttgart, and Hamburg were generously given 50 percent of the ovine death rate on Gruinard. A hundred bomblets clustered in a 500 pound RAF bomb were calculated to riddle with anthrax 10 acres of town or 50 acres in the country. Four thousand 500 pound scatter bombs would do for Stuttgart, 40,350 would finish off the lot, with Aachen and Wilhelmshaven thrown in as a bonus. The 4,000,000 bomblets would be spattered by 2,690 bomber-sorties, easily achieved by an air force that a year later could put 1,000 planes over Cologne in a night.

Churchill was impressed with the scheme. Anthrax was admittedly not cricket, but neither was the war. Any night the church bells of Sussex and Kent might peal the official warning that the Wehrmacht had set jackboot on English shingle. Besides, we needed a tit-for-tat, in case the unspeakable Hitler decided to save himself shot and shell by spraying anthrax all over *us*. The anthrax missile went into production.

This was tricky. A tragic mishap filling the usual sort of bomb meant the end of a factory and perhaps a hundred war workers. With anthrax bomblets, a slip-up was liable in time to decimate the British population.

Then came Pearl Harbor. The might of American ingenuity was unleashed against the dictators (not the Russian one, who had changed sides). While American laboratories poured out penicillin in a flood unimaginable to the British—who were growing it in bedpans and milk churns in the animal house of the pathology school in Oxford—the U.S. Chemical Warfare Service equally efficiently started popping out anthrax bomblets. Berlin, Stuttgart, Frankfurt, Hamburg, Aachen, and Wilhelmshaven, they assured their British allies, would be fully taken care of by the Yanks.

Like many of Churchill's clever conceptions—the mighty Hukkabuk floating forts made from ice and wood chips, the oil pipes to set the sea ablaze in 1940 and boil the Germans—the anthrax project saw service no more active than the generals sitting comfortably in Whitehall and the Pentagon. Time is as unkind to man's inventions as to man himself. The glittering technology of one year is the scrap-heap of the next. The luxurious *Queen Mary* was ousted by the jet, the chatter of the radio by the glare of TV, canned peas became frozen, and the backs of envelopes capitulated to the pocket calculator. The murderous inheritance of the anthrax bomb was cruelly usurped by the atom bomb.

Anthrax retained its devotees, like those enthusiasts who puff passionately for steam-trains, or race to Brighton in vintage cars. They included Brigadier O. H. Wansbrough-Jones, who wrote to the Chief of Staffs with charming optimism in 1945, "Its use in minor wars on which it is not worth using atom bombs, or major ones in which they were being barred, is not impossible."

### Reasons for Dropping the Atom Rather Than the Anthrax Bomb.

1. The population of Berlin, Stuttgart, Frankfurt, Hamburg, Aachen, and Wilhelmshaven could be reasonably reliably exterminated by six 1945 atom bombs (possibly only five, Frankfurt and Stuttgart being near enough to share). This would need only six Flying Fortress sorties, not 2,690 Lancaster sorties.
2. Though the anthrax bomb is considerably quieter, a big bang impresses the enemy tremendously.
3. Anthrax fallout cannot be easily measured with a Geiger counter.
4. An atom bomb is probably easier to make, is easier to handle, and looks better.
5. Death from an atomic explosion occurs in a millisecond, with anthrax you have to wait a week.
6. The atom bomb is more warlike. Nobody ever got a medal for spreading disease.

It is fascinating to speculate on the course of world history had Hiroshima been attacked on August 6, 1945, with 1,000 tons of anthrax instead.

That summer, man stood amid the rotting bones of his own inhumanity. The horrors exhumed by the allied armies were so widespread and terrible, everyone forgot about the sacrificial sheep of Gruinard. Except Dr. Fildes, who had thereby become Sir Paul.

Everyone had also forgotten about the spores. They could lie like murderous Sleeping Beauties in the soil for years. The British Government had forgotten its own Anthrax Order of 1938, decreeing that animals dead from anthrax should be instantly buried on the spot in quicklime, like its executed murderers. At the end of World War II, on September 2, 1945, the only dangerous place left in Europe was Gruinard Island.

On the mainland, braw men gazed upon it for years and shook

timorously over the drams, like kilted Translyvanians around Dracula's castle. Mothers threatened misbehaving bairns with maroonment. The minister preached against it, when he was temporarily short of other evil.

A large black-and-white metal notice now warns from the shore:

GRUINARD ISLAND
THIS ISLAND IS GOVERNMENT PROPERTY THE GROUND IS CONTAMINATED AND DANGEROUS LANDING IS PRO-HIBITED BY ORDER 1966.

This gentle little island, a perch for sea birds, a haven for fish, has like Bikini Atoll been condemned by mankind to solitude for geological life. Worse medical disasters have occurred, but not on Gruinard. It ruined the tourist trade.

On short summer nights when the breeze comes lightly from the northwest, they say you can hear the plaintive, baaing, coughing of anthrax-infected sheep.

# 31

## SUFFER THE LITTLE CHILDREN
### *If Politically Advantageous*

In 1971 a Tory Minister of Education abolished the free milk that schoolchildren had been imbibing each noon since the Battle of Britain, or possibly Agincourt.

Every country has its explosive political conjunctions. In Germany, Nazi and past. In France, minister and mistress. In Italy, mayor and Mafia.

In Britain, it is children and milk.

Labour was outraged, unbelieving, furious. It saddled the Tories with transmuting the burgeoning generation into a sickly pack of wizened midgets. The Tories thought the money should be spent on something useful, like books.

Merthyr Tydfil in the green valleys of South Wales had the tenderest regard for little children, or one of the heftiest Labour parliamentary majorities in the country. Putting humanity before mortification, its town council voted to defy the Queen's writ and went on delivering the milk of human kindness. Martyrdom lasted a month, until the borough treasurer refused to sign checks for the dairy.

The Merthyr Tydfil council eyed aghast its bright-eyed, lilting-voiced youngsters, who would perish without milk as surely as premature infants in their incubators. The effect on Welsh rugby football was unthinkable. They tremblingly let "regardless of their doom, The little victims play." The doom was documented seven years later by the Medical Research Council in Cardiff.

The doctors followed 581 Welsh 8-year-olds, all with three or more brothers and sisters, 571 of them from "working-class" families, 134 with fathers on welfare, and 46 from the socially infamous single-parent families.

Half had milk every schoolday, half not. The milk-drinking boys became averagely 0.11 centimeters shorter, and 0.21 kilograms fatter, the girls 0.45 centimeters taller and 0.05 kilograms fatter—figures which "do not achieve statistical significance.... The re-introduction of free school milk for 7-11-year-old children is unlikely to have any appreciable effect on the physical development of the children."

In 1974 mercy returned to British politics with another Labour government. Its Minister of Education, Mrs. Shirley Williams, restored free school milk despite the Minister of Health imploring her not to. The milk was offered cut-rate by the European Economic Community, which has the compassion toward little ones of the Merthyr Tydfil town council and an enormous milk surplus.

The fatter the milk the fatter the EEC subsidy, which made the Coronary Prevention Group furious. *Over*nutrition is now our children's problem, and the poor little things will all drop dead from heart attacks at age 30. The British genius for compromise is being directed toward skim milk.

Politically, you cannot tell milk from lead. Whether lead turns your children into shambling morons depends on your vote. The humanitarian Labour party is committed headlong to expunging lead from gasoline. The Tories are more wary of the scientists' conflicting reports. Of 166 children living near a London lead-works, those with a low lead-level were found to be more scholastically accomplished. But they were 16 months older than the high lead-level ones. Besides, many Tory voters have oil shares in their portfolios. Pornography has a similar effect on the brain to lead, seen from different political poles. Tobacco emits Calverley's sublime fragrance for its workers' union, and nuclear annihilation seems not nearly so bad if you are a right-winger.

Politicians' inability to respond rationally to proven facts is frightening, but the papers would be disastrously dull without it.

Stopping the milk did not retard the career of the Tory minister, who was Mrs. Thatcher.

# 32

## DISASTROUS DISASTERS
### *Trop de Zèle*

At 3 A.M. on a morning in February 1976, there was an earthquake in Guatemala. It killed 23,000 and injured 75,000. The world gasped, wrung its hands, and poured aid upon the stricken Central Americans.

UNDRO, CARE, CRS, and OFDA hit them like intercontinental missiles (United Nations Disaster Relief Organization, Cooperative for American Relief Everywhere, Catholic Relief Service, U.S. Office of Foreign Disaster Assistance). CARE and CRS rushed the Guatemalians 25,000 tons of food. The Guatemalians were not short of food. The local corn lost a third of its price. The local farmers were ruined.

One hundred and fifteen tons of drugs arrived instantly. These included contraceptives, some mysterious tablets made in 1934, tranquilizers, blood pressure-reducing drugs, and assorted sample packs for American physicians. Three Guatemalian pharmacists tried sorting them out, but after three months bulldozed a hole and buried them.

Doctors appeared by the planeload, with a prefabricated hospital. None spoke Spanish. The local doctors and nurses were ravenously devouring the work, in a week their hospitals were operating normally. The American hospital was nevertheless erected and treated patients, at $70,000 for each.

There was an earthquake at Lice, Turkey, in 1975. Oxfam hurried 419 polyurethane temporary houses, erected them in 60 days. Two days earlier, the Turkish government had finished 1,500 permanent relief houses, everyone was busy housewarming.

In 1974 the Ethiopian Relief Commission raised the alarm. If the rains failed again there would be terrible famine in the south. There was already appalling famine in the north. Nobody took any notice. A disaster about to happen is as little news as a dog possibly going to bite a man. A disaster needs photographs of starving black babies, howling widows, and legless men to make it box-office.

The Ethiopian famine arrived as promised. The United Nations created camps to feed the nomadic victims, and killed many of them with diseases to which their isolated life left them susceptible.

People do not all panic, go mad, flee like lemmings after disasters. Not all disasters bring horrific epidemics, despite photographs of clean white doctors and nurses sticking needles into everyone in sight. All disaster-struck governments are not corrupt. Food may be scattered but not destroyed. Nobody loses all their clothes or all their friends. "Experts have not been able to trace a single recorded death from exposure after a disaster," the London *Sunday Times* reported, "even in extremely cold conditions."

When up against raw Nature, man intelligently improvises. Otherwise, he would never have evolved to enjoy the comforts that competing relief agencies hustle so haphazardly to restore.

# 33

## THE DYING ART
### *Hamfisted Hangmen*

A dwindling posse of nations arms itself with judicial killing, but the scaffold is not yet a piece of incomprehensible furniture. The House of Commons was still debating it in 1982. Enthusiasts and abhorrers should be clear what they argue about. What could put it plainer than Sir Sydney Smith's *Forensic Medicine*?

> The execution is carried out as follows:
>
> The prisoner is placed on a platform above trap doors which open downwards when a bolt is drawn. A rope is looped around the neck with the knot under the angle of the jaw and with a sufficient length of rope to allow a drop of 5 to 7 feet according to the weight of the person.
>
> On pulling the bolt the condemned individual drops to the length of the rope; the sudden stoppage of the moving body associated with the position of the knot causes the head to be jerked violently, dislocating or fracturing the cervical column and rupturing the cord. The dislocation often takes place between the second and third cervical vertebrae. Death is instantaneous, although the heart may continue to beat for several minutes. This method of execution is very expeditious and cleanly.
>
> The postmortem appearances are of no consequence.

According to Sir Sydney, hanging is as efficient as tooth pulling and sounds less harmful.

Even inhumanity is bedeviled by human error. In the 1890s, Mr. Berry, a breezy Yorkshireman whose hobby was otter-hunting, was the Escoffier, the Pavlova, the Lord Lister of hanging. He brought style and science to the scaffold. He invented a formula to calculate the drop (aiming at a striking force of 24 hundredweight) and assessed each victim's neck tissues with the assiduousness of a throat surgeon.

Even Homer sometimes nods and so did this Homeric hangman. He failed with Mr. John Lee. The subject's joy was tempered by Mr. Berry's immediate attempt to rectify his error by stringing him up again twice in succession. On November 30, 1895, Mr. Robert Goodale's head was jerked off at Norwich Castle, but the coroner excused Mr. Berry for only a slip in his arithmetic. He almost pulled another one off in Liverpool on August 29, 1891, Mr. John Conway's, but that was the fault of heeding the prison doctor, who was pushing his own pamphlet, *Judicial Hanging*.

Less academic hangmen of the nineteenth century faced messier results. The disappearance through the trap in Durham of Mr. Matthew Atkinson, a local miner, was followed by a dull thud below and a snapped rope above. He had nothing worse than a dislocated jaw, and it took twenty-four minutes before they could rig everything up and hang him again.

Mr. John Coffey suffered the same mishap and was retrieved from the pit with blood spurting from his ears. The rope annoyingly broke again, but someone neatly caught him before he hit bottom. The third time they strangled him and it took twelve minutes—one hour and one minute less than needed for Mr. Antonio Sprecage in Canada.

With Mr. Patrick Harnet, "a heavy gurgling sound was heard, and soon the blood in torrents commenced pouring on the stone floor below." Hangman Marwood—with whom Mr. Berry enjoyed the relationship of brilliant intern to senior surgeon—dropped Mr. Brownless too far and embedded a one-and-a-half inch rope in his neck, blood everywhere. (This also occurred in Durham, a city to be avoided for murder.) Mr. Berry himself shuddered at anything thicker than three-quarters of an inch, comprising five strands of silky Italian hemp, four strands for women.

The executioner of four men in a British colony in 1927 was in a hurry to go and hang some more, so he did them in pairs. The surgeon discovered one groaning and gasping after his hasty departure. All four bodies were suspended for another fifteen minutes, just to make sure.

It was murmured that the last woman hanged in Britain needed a burly warder to score success with a rugby football tackle. Expert hands have now lost their art with disuse, like fan-painters. The natural extinction of the professional hangman is surely the best argument for his abolition. What is worth doing at all is worth doing well.

Energetic, imaginative American scientific ingenuity, which gave the world anesthesia, provided also electrocution. The advantages were obvious—no danger of the head coming off, it would be nice for the subject to sit down, the chance of a snapped rope was greater than a blown fuse. Only spoilsports suggest that the legal 2,000 volts just stuns, death coming from the legal postmortem immediately afterward. Mr. William Kemmler blazed the trail on August 6, 1890 at Auburn, N.Y.

The modern guillotine was equally convenient. You stepped up to a board like a pier mirror, in the fresh air (and before an admiring audience until recently), were securely strapped, smoothly tipped to the horizontal, secured with a stout wooden collar, *et violà*!

This great labor-saving device was invented by Dr. Joseph-Ignace Guillotin on October 10, 1789. He was anxious that *égalité* should enjoy its logical conclusion. Like other social events in Europe, public executions were plagued by snobbery. Nobles were decapitated, the rabble hanged. The aristocrats took beheading seriously. It would never do to lose their dignity as well. The second queen who King Henry VIII sent to the block spent the night before rehearsing.

The prototype guillotine was painstakingly tested with live sheep and dead people, and at 3:30 P.M. on April 25, 1792, M. Nicholas-Jacques Pelletier incited its maiden drop in the Place de Grève. The machine quickly appeared as toys, souvenirs, earrings. It caught public fancy like the yo-yo.

Unlike hanging and electrocution, where the heart trips on

merrily for minutes, you were blatantly dead when bundled, in two pieces, into the long wicker box like a music-hall artiste's wardrobe trunk.

Or were you?

"An old *surveillant* at St. Jean," wrote Somerset Maugham, "tells a story of how a doctor had arranged with a man who was to be guillotined to blink three times if he could after his head was cut off, and says he saw him blink twice."

Dr. Frederick Gaertner recounted another disastrous defiance. "Immediately after the head was severed and dropped in the basket, I took charge of it. The facial expression was that of great agony, for several minutes after decapitation. He would open his eyes, also his mouth, in the process of gaping, as if he wanted to speak to me, and I am positive he could see me for several seconds after the head was severed from the body. There is no doubt that the brain was still active."

Dr. Velpeau in 1864 invited his professional brother, Dr. de la Pommerais, who he was going to watch being guillotined in the morning, to blink his right eye three times afterward in response to his shouted name, but he could manage only once. The head of 24-year-old Charlotte Corday, who four days before had murdered Dr. Jean-Paul Marat in his bath, blushed indignantly when displayed to the mob. A medical student stuck a scalpel into a newly detached head and produced a grimace. A head tossed into a sack with another bit it. Some corpses ran around for ten minutes like headless chickens.

On November 13, 1879, three doctors were driven by these tales to experiment on 23-year-old M. Théotime Prunier, shouting in his detached face, sticking in pins, applying ammonia under his nose, silver nitrate and candle flames to his eyeballs. Only response, "The face bore a look of astonishment."

Gassing is less accident prone, but miserably unspectacular. The guillotine, while it remained on offer, was probably the preferable enforcement of a premature end. There was always the outside chance you could spit in your executioner's eye.

# Part Seven

# THE QUICK
# AND THE DEAD

# 34

## A TOUCH OF CLASS

### *Waiting Room Disaster*

In 1661, Charles II granted a charter to the Royal Society for Improving Natural Knowledge (a founder member was Sir Christopher Wren). He contributed valuably to medical science by increasing the annual ration of hanged criminals for dissection by the Royal College of Surgeons from four to six. He was simultaneously the biggest buff among English monarchs for the Royal Touch to cure the King's Evil (scrofula, swollen tuberculous glands of the neck). This worked as the touch of God, percolated through the divine right of kings. It was performed ceremoniously with choirs, beefeaters, and ladies and gentlemen in waiting. Charles treated 92,107 patients, the rush was once so great that six were trampled to death.

# 35

## BEACHY HEAD

### *Preventive Medicine Breakthrough*

The South Downs fall into the English Channel at Beachy Head, a sheer cliff 532 feet high, pure chalk, gleaming in the sun like an actress's smile.

To the east nestles the seemly Sussex resort of Eastbourne, largely owned by the Duke of Devonshire. Its small white hotels edge a Marine Parade on which pale, wizened people sit in deck chairs reading Agatha Christie—like the sand in an hourglass, the population sinks to the bottom of Britain as it ages, in the pathetic hope that the weather might be a little better. The Bell Tout lighthouse was built atop the Head in 1831, the British and Dutch fleet were beaten there by the French on June 30, 1690, the British admiral was courtmartialled.

What the Bernese Oberland is to serious skiers, Beachy Head is to resolute suicides.

People were falling over Beachy Head before St. Augustine arrived along the coast at Thanet to convert the Anglo-Saxons in 596. Two or three a year dropped off during this century, reaching a steady average of four in 1965. Like other well-publicized open-air activities, the participants recently steadily increased. In 1971 ten went over, in 1976 sixteen, in 1979 twelve.

You can commit suicide by diving headfirst from your bedroom window. If choosing 532 feet gives the opportunity of changing your mind while in transit, there is nothing you can do about it. The disastrous fascination of Beachy Head as a springboard for shuffling off this mortal coil is complex.

British Rail runs an excellent hourly service from London's Victoria Station, and the expense of a return ticket is avoided. (Three out of four suicidal tumblers travel from inland Britain, five in the last twenty years came specially from abroad to do it.) Jumping off Beachy Head runs in some families. One suicide generally brings the next within a fortnight, another example of man's infinite suggestibility and lack of originality.

The most popular months are July and August (19 each), March and June (13). April is the cruelest month nationally for self-destruction, but drops only three at Beachy Head. Friday is the favorite day, indicating that not everybody lives for the weekend. The busiest spot is by the new under-cliff lighthouse (23 in fifteen years). The White Cliffs of Dover have only one suicide a year, but the summer bus schedules up Beachy Head are better.

Not everyone you see hurtling from Beachy Head is committing suicide. Cliffs are dangerous places for romping, bird-nesting, or seeking sexual seclusion. There are accepted indications that the fall was intentional—a woman wandering away from her hand-bag, a man neatly folding his overcoat or gulping a bottle of whisky or shouting to look out down below or making a graceful swan dive. One taxi driver reflected too late on the fare who directed him there from the gates of a psychiatric hospital.

The grisly record of *felo de se* has brilliantly been stayed. Since 1975 the suicide rate at Beachy Head has been halved. This was achieved with no elaborate construction work, no complicated surveillance, and at no additional public expense. They changed the local coroner.

The new man needed stronger persuasion that his subjects *intended* to topple over the grassy edge. The whisky drinkers, for instance, were given the benefit of being in no condition to decide clearly one way or another. From twenty Beach Head deaths in 1965-69, 65 percent were suicides. From 65 deaths in 1975-79, only 32 percent were, a drop in ten years of 33 percent.

This is a sensational advance in preventive medicine. Deaths from cancer had meanwhile *increased* by some 10 percent, from heart disease by 5 percent. A comparable triumph was the elimination of polio by prophylaxis with Salk vaccine.

Happily for mankind, the Beachy Head principle is being adopted to wider medicine. Any cause of death is a matter of honest opinion. The Royal College of Physicians of London claim that one-fifth of British death certificates give an incorrect reason, and a quarter contain other errors. Birmingham and Edinburgh, more advanced in research, have achieved a 40 percent inaccuracy.

This method has already eradicated cholera from several small tropical nations, putting it down as death from summer diarrhea. In the distant, icy winter of 1939, medical officers prevented a humiliating epidemic of German measles in the British army by reporting it as spots with a bad cold. The frightening new diseases that pour from research wards—Marfan's disease, Marchiafava-Michaeli syndrome, antiglomerular basement membrane antibody nephritis, and the like—will thankfully be swiftly eliminated, because those family doctors who have heard of them will anyway be incapable of recognizing them.

Most people die in the hospital from the Beachy Head syndrome. Elderly patients have so many diseases, the intern puzzles which to put first. If he mentions the fall from a bicycle that brought the patient to hospital six months ago, there will be endless fuss with the coroner. If he mentions "alcoholism" he will outrage the relatives. If he mentions "postoperative shock" he will outrage the surgeon. If he seeks advice, consultants are as unexcited about their dead patients as actors about their closed shows.

After playing the diagnoses like patience, the intern generally selects bronchopneumonia—"the old man's friend" of pre-antibiotic medicine—signs the death certificate, and collects his ash cash (extra fee from cremation). It is a kindly laxity to diagnose for the dying diseases that are familiar and respectable. The patients can succumb to them in saintly resignation.

# Part Eight

# A Dictionary
# of Disaster

# 36

## IT'S A CRUEL WORLD

### *Disastrous A-Z*

A Wodehouseian telegram once read:

COME AT ONCE DISASTER STARES FACE.

It does, everywhere. The mildest man, the wariest woman, need barely venture from garden gate, office desk, or factory bench to risk Nature's subtle thunderbolts.

### *Asbestos*

Greek for "inextinguishable." Emits microscopic fibers of mineral silicates, which, when inhaled, turn the lung from a sponge to a suet pudding. Symptoms can take 25 years to appear, half the patients later develop lung cancer. The Mount Sinai School of Medicine in New York calculates that someone in the U.S.A. will die from this complication every 50 minutes until the end of the century. Affects dockers, boilermen, pipe-laggers, demolition workers, makers of brake linings, and the wives washing their overalls. The gas masks issued to the entire British population in September 1938 (Munich) had asbestos filters, could have done Hitler's job for him.

## Bees

Every year bees and wasps kill one in ten million among the population of Britain, Western Europe, and the United States. This is more than killed by atomic energy, but causes less fuss.

## Calories

Toward the end of this century, books on calories proliferate like those on Christianity toward the end of the last. They are similarly severe or sympathetic, fearsome or fanciful, logical or lunatic, and as feebly effective in producing either holiness or slimness. A disastrous waste of money. Two words are enough to lose weight—*eat less*.

## Dogs

Doggy Black Death is romping toward the Channel. A rabies epidemic that started in Poland spread through Germany and Switzerland, a third of France is now officially infested, the foxes have got it at Cherbourg. Europe had 19,549 rabid animals in 1981, a rise of a quarter in four years. Foxes suffered most, 13,262 of them. Dogs, 1,770. Dogs are dangerous for ten days before they start foaming at the mouth. A bitten human can spend a year nervously waiting for the disease to appear.

## Expectations

The life expectancy of a newborn male has risen from 48.1 years in 1901 to 69.8 in the 1980s, a bonus of 21 years and the next summer. This seems a superb achievement of our brilliant doctors and visionary politicians, who have made the world so glorious for hypochondria and bureaucracy. The statistics are disastrously misleading. The diseases of middle age still kill. A man of 40—just beginning to enjoy himself with a Mercedes and a mistress—has an increased life since 1910 of only 5.6 years. Aged 50, of 3.7. Aged 70, barely from one Christmas to the next. Women live 6 years longer than men. Those women so earnest about equality should consider extending it to the mortality rates.

### Fungi

The Death Cap toadstool (*Amanita Phalloides*) causes 90 percent of deaths from fungus poisoning. You see it in the woods all summer, dirty-white satiny cap, white gills, white ring dangling from stem and ragged sheath rising from foot. It is readily confused with an edible mushroom. The antidote is known to Dr. Pierre Bastien in Remieremont, a small town in the Vosges, who ate them sautéed in butter on television to prove it. The False Death Cap (Amanita citrina) is similar, but smells of raw potato. It may be eaten with impunity. It is best not to try.

### Glue

Modern glues are disastrously disruptive to law and order. Their inhaled solvents produce hallucinations, addiction, death. And this sort of thing happens:

"A prisoner and his wife were taken to hospital from a courtroom in Gloucestershire after binding themselves together with superglue. Edward S...., aged 27, had been remanded in custody for a week on an assault charge when his wife Wendy, aged 25, entered a detention room with the glue on her palms. They locked hands and police could not tear them apart. The couple were taken to the Gloucestershire Royal Hospital, where doctors prised them apart." (See Chapter 37, Love Locked In.)

### Home

For disaster, there's no place like it. Most accidents happen at home. Over 500 British children under five are killed at home every year—choking on playthings, suffocating in plastic bags, scalding themselves in the kitchen, falling downstairs and into the fire, poisoning themselves with grownups' pretty drug tablets. The tragedy of these tragedies is that with parental foresight and commonsense most are preventable.

### Iatrogenesis

Greek for "caused by physicians." The public has known for centuries that hospitals are dangerous places. University Hospital, Boston, Massachusetts, has proved it. Of 815 patients there, 290 were suffering from the effects of their treatment, 76 seriously so, and 15 were shortly killed by it. Modern doctors are prodigal with drugs and tests. This is partly from admirable conscientiousness, partly from terror of being sued for negligence, partly because in many countries they come completely free (except for their taxpayers). But mostly because these risky remedies and hazardous investigations allow patients to scrape through a succession of previously fatal illnesses.

## Jail

A frightful thing happened at Cambridge in 1522. His Majesty's judge, gorgeously robed, convened with lawyers in wigs and gowns, brilliantly uniformed sheriffs, the University vice-chancellor in academicals, the chaplain in canonicals, the mayor in full municipal panoply, the trumpeters, criers, and pikemen. They were trying the wretches delivered clanking from the county jails, flogging, branding, and hanging them, that they might reform their wicked ways. The prisoners exacted terrible revenge. All were jumping with lice, which carry typhus fever (there was a lot of it about in the sixteenth century). "Jail fever" was an accepted part of your punishment, like the bread and water. The lice jumped from bar to bench, infected the judicial pageant and perfectly respectable people throughout the town. The "Black Assizes" was repeated at Oxford in 1577, killing 510 people, and at Exeter in 1589, decimating Devon. You are unlikely to catch typhus in the splendidly appointed jails of the West, but it is another reason for behaving yourself in the USSR.

## Kippers

Disaster broke over the two-faced head of this succulent breakfast for the English gentleman. Egalitarian Americans ungentlemanly discovered that kippers gave you cancer. It was the hydrocarbons from the smoking. So did barbecued steaks, forked from the glowing griddle by your genial ginned-up host, resembling what they used to rake from the boilers of steamships. The Americans later relented. You needed to eat a shoal of kippers a

week, and go to barbecues for life. The only remote danger a
kipper presents to the English gentleman is choking on one of its
innumerable bones through seeing something funny in *The
Times*.

## Legionnaires

Legionnaires' disease is pneumonia caused by a germ that
stays at the best hotels. It was named from a disastrous outbreak
at the American Legion Convention at Philadelphia in 1976. The
illness has an honorable military ring, even a shimmering suggestion of *Beau Geste*. It could as easily have been Elks' disease,
Buffaloes' disease, Bar Association disease, Medical Association
disease or Morticians' disease.

## Melancholy

Worry is bad for your health. What do the British worry about
most? Their health. Forty percent in 1982, compared with 14
percent in 1951. Thirty years ago, there was much less health to
worry about—no heart transplants, cigarettes never gave you
cancer nor butter a coronary, neither battered wives nor jogging
had yet been invented. Ninety-nine percent of Britons award
health the greatest value in life. A gloomily prosaic view, rein-
forced by food and drink at 82 percent, running well clear of
sexual relations at 72 percent.

## Nature

"If the substances which mother nature puts into our foods
were to be judged as critically as those items which man adds, we
might soon find the safety of many common foods questioned."
The British Nutrition Foundation shudders over cabbages, broad
beans, turnips, rhubarb, homemade jam, and the potato, which
contains 150 different chemicals, including arsenic. The addi-
tives that so upset health-food enthusiasts make manufactured
foods *safer*. Without chemical preservatives, urbanized countries
would suffer dull diets or starvation. White sugar is the purest of
foods, but condemned as impure by the purists because it is so

refined. Butter is called nature's food, margarine man's. When both have enjoyed the marvels of food technology, they bear little resemblance to their original milk or vegetable oil. The sensational difference between free-range chickens and battery hens, between compost-grown wholemeal loaf stone-ground by the Friends of the Earth and the sliced stuff from supermarkets, between sunflower seeds and sausages, is the higher prices that nature charges in the health shops.

## Oranges

A London girl aged 15 used her teeth to unscrew the metal cap on a plastic bottle of orange juice. It had fermented during two months outside a refrigerator and blew up. She arrived in hospital pouring blood from her mouth. The surgeons could see down her throat the bared, pulsating left carotid artery—had this been severed, death from exsanguination or from suffocation would have been an academic point. She recovered, but her tonsils had been avulsed. It was no compensation for the poor girl to be the only case in surgical history of tonsillectomy performed by explosive.

## Pot

Marijuana gives you food poisoning. The Center for Disease Control in Atlanta found 85 young adults infected with exactly the same variety of *Salmonella* germ. This would usually indicate eating in the same dirty restaurant, but the victims were scattered across the United States. All smoked pot. The supply of each was found rich in *Salmonella* bacteria. This lives in the gut. It came from animal faeces applied either as a fertilizer or a profitable adulterant. Enough to put you off drugs for life.

## Queers

Male homosexuals risk a hurtful selection of diseases. Syphilis is transmitted more commonly homosexually. They catch gonorrhoea and lymphogranuloma, like heterosexuals. They become infected with protozoa—primitive one-cell organisms—including the *Entamoeba histolytica* bringing amoebic dysentry and liver abscess. Protozoa combined with the fashionable cytomegalovirus—which can be sexually transmitted—produces serious lung disease. They are also liable to hepatitis B (the nasty one). There is a lot of sadness in being gay.

### Risks

*A Risk Ready Reckoner.* Driving a car for 4,000 miles = the same risk as smoking 100 cigarettes = 2 hours rock climbing = 1 year working in the chemical industry. The risk of riding a motorbike for 350 hours = 16 hours a day at home for 2 years (see HOME) = drinking 40 bottles of wine = eating 80 jars of peanut butter. A nuclear power accident killing 1,000 = same risk as dams, coalmines, ships, railways (see BEES). Magically removing all other causes of death, a steelworker doing 2,000 hours a year would live to be 6,000, a man driving a car 10 hours a week would die aged 3,500, riding a motorbike aged only 300. Anyone smoking 40 cigarettes a day would just make 100. Professor Trevor Kletz of Loughborough University says so.

### Sheep

The English Lake District, Welsh valleys, and Scottish glens are best avoided. Sheep are dangerous animals. In conspiracy with man's best friend, deadly. The dog eats infected sheepmeat, develops in its gut the *Echinococcus granulosus* tapeworm (4 mm long, 4 suckers, and 40 hooklets), passes the egg in its feces, and infects a human, who may end with a cyst in liver or lungs the size of a football. Sheep thus caused seven deaths in 1979, more than snakes.

### Tights

The second female curse (cystitis) spread during the 1960s with the miniskirt and the substitution of tights for stockings-and-garter belts. The close-fitting nylon invited infection by retaining moisture and heat while excluding air. Also, tights were such a bother to get down, the ladies peed much less frequently.

### Urea

Pump urea formaldehyde foam into wall cavities: it sets hard, insulates the home, and admirably furthers Western policies by conserving energy. It also emits pungent formaldehyde gas (so do anatomists' corpses), causing weeping, vomiting, chest pains. After complaints from 2,000 retching householders, the U.S. Consumer Product Safety Commission banned it. The problem is different in Britain, most houses being of brick. The minerals in bricks emit 30 times the radiation of a nuclear power station. You pay a mortgage on them, too.

### Video

The 17-year-old daughter of a Bristol video games engineer played with them two hours a day in his workshop. Space Invader, Asteroids, Space Fury, Defender, Lunar Rescue, no trouble. With Dark Warrior, she collapsed. Distraught father imagined her electrocuted, rushed her to hospital. She was sensitive to the multicolored flashing lights, the first case of Dark Warrior epilepsy. A young Rumanian had previously suffered Astro Fighter epilepsy. You also can get a sprained wrist from them.

### Water

Getting drunk on water is more disastrous than on alcohol—swelling of the brain, convulsions, coma, death. Anyone can suffer water intoxication, from drinking too much water too quickly. Far better stick to gin.

### Xmas

Our busiest season for self-destruction runs from the primroses to the roses. In bleak midwinter, the suicide rate slackens.

Perhaps the chill cheerlessness of the world hardly merits drastic release from it. The exception is Christmas. The effect of the festive season on a man confined to his home with his relatives for a week of dyspepsia and awful hangovers is plainly disastrous. The National Institute for Mental Health at Bethesda, Maryland, suggests a subtler cause, the "gray sky syndrome." Some people during the short days crave to hibernate, like the bears. They suffer loss of energy (including sexual), gloom, and anxiety. The treatment is fluorescent lighting throughout the home, automatically turned on and off at midsummer sunrise and sunset. Fine, but it will make the house plants dreadfully neurotic.

### Youth

Many people would like to be rather richer, and when they are would like to be rather younger. The one can lead to the other, they imagine. Early this century, Russian Professor Serge Voronoff rounded up some doddery and threadbare rams, grafted the testicles of young ones, and had them leaping like lambs. He went to Paris with the idea of trying it on humans, but encountered deplorable lack of philanthropy among young men over giving up their testicles to old ones. Nor were the authorities receptive to a spin-off from the guillotine, blade falling at both ends. Voronoff used apes instead. In the 1920s his "monkey gland" treatment made him as famous as Charlie Chaplin. The professor grew rich, and if his patients grew no younger they faced life more hopefully than the monkeys. The disastrous effects of seeking youth were displayed in an elaborate *Punch* cartoon of 1925, showing an elderly lady addicted to rejuvenating tonic ending up twelve drawings later as a heap of baby clothes.

### Zeal

As fatally disastrous in medical men as in military ones.

# Part Nine

# SEXUAL ENTRAPMENTS

# 37

# LOVE LOCKED IN

## Dubious Disaster

The film *What's Up Nurse?* had an amorous couple on British Rail who got jammed, in the loo. Note comma.

Amid flashing blue lights, shrieking sirens, and scarlet blankets, they sped for surgical disentanglement. This operation is as fictional as the penis transplant in *Percy,* the movie which did better business in its native Britain than *The Sound of Music.*

Penis captivus was well known in the Middle Ages. It was God's punishment for copulating among the owls and bats in night-shrouded churches and churchyards. Release was effected at cockcrow, by prayers and buckets of cold water.

The first case recorded by a doctor was in 1729, the next in 1923 at Warsaw, in the park. The couple were so ashamed when it got in the papers, they shot themselves.

*The Sexual Life of Our* [1908] *Time* describes another in Bremen docks. "A great crowd assembled, from the midst of which the unfortunate couple were removed in a closed carriage, and taken to the hospital, and not until chloroform had been administered to the girl did the spasm pass off and free the man." For another case, two years later, they had to crack ice as well.

Furtive fornication in the open air was blamed. Nervous contraction of powerful muscles around the vagina trapped the erect penis, like a sailing-ship in a bottle. Such fearsome spasm was powerfully augmented by the rapid gathering of a crowd not sympathetically inclined to the girl's blushes.

It was not always a vicious vice. It could clamp in the marriage bed. One new wife in the 1860s suffered treatment "which involved the application of a probe, speculum, compressive sponge, glycerine tampons etc. . . . This young and chronically neurotic woman grew every week more agitated and excitable so that she eventually responded to the smallest aggravation with compulsive crying fits."

Her husband bravely tried a cure through a natural application, and escaped with bruises.

The captive penis has not arisen this century. Cases of foreskin hooked on an intrauterine device like a rising trout do not count. Penis captivus is perhaps as much a mythical Victorian disease as clergyman's sore throat or scriveners' palsy. Should it strike on the back seat of your Fiesta, it is best to blow down each others' nostrils. It seems to work with horses.

# 38

## BREAKING IT OFF
### *Liberated Female Disaster*

Prolonged intercourse, particularly with the female subject in the superior position, and inadvertent flexion of the erect penis are well described cases of penile trauma commonly leading to corporeal rupture.

—*Journal of Urology*

# 39

## THE MOST UNKINDEST CUT OF ALL

### *Vasectomy Vagaries*

I have treated no patients for thirty years, but am regularly solicited for medical advice at parties and picnics, across dinner tables and bars, and by people overhearing me called "Doctor" in the line at the bank or the butcher's. Once, signing my works in a classy London bookshop, I was interrupted by a clergyman pulling up his somber trouser leg and inviting inspection of his knee. He explained you had to wait so long at the doctor's office. Perhaps patients prefer consulting me, because any disagreeable advice carries no moral obligation of its acceptance, or even belief.

One case I can diagnose on its approach with vodka-and-tonic in hand. A man under thirty with a low-handicap look, who volunteers that the two kids are fine, but they're changing the Volvo for a Datsun and it's Florida this summer not Ibiza, and there's all this in the papers about the pill, why not end the fretting and fussing at a stroke, well two strokes, I'm thinking seriously about a vasectomy, Doc, what would you advise me to do?

Vasectomy is the securest contraceptive next to abstinence. Sterilization knows no equality—the failure rate is 0.02 percent for men, 0.13 percent for women. The pill has a failure rate of 0.16 percent, intrauterine devices of 1.5 percent, foaming chemicals of

11.9 percent, the condom of 3.6 percent, coitus interruptus of 6.7 percent, and the rhythm method a discordant 15.5 percent.

A vasectomy is also a declaration of marital adherence more solemn than anything uttered at the altar.

The cut lifeline is the vas deferens, a muscular-walled tube conveying sperm from the testicle to the world at large. It runs through hernia country. The surgeon can feel a hard thread among the small arteries, veins, and nerves composing the spermatic cord. These strands are wrapped in the filmy cremaster muscle, performer of the cremasteric reflex, a tautening on the testes in response to someone delicately stroking the inner thigh. This is more agreeable, if the circumstances are right, than having your knee-jerks hammered.

Vasectomy is as fashionable an ingredient of active, modern male life as skin diving, windsurfing and hang-gliding. It was being performed in the days of hansom cabs and the bustle. "This treatment is already obsolescent," the *Theory and Practice of Surgery* dismissed the operation in 1903. They tried it to shrink enlarged prostates, but the patients "have rapidly aged or become demented from this loss, it has been conjectured, of the stimulating influence of testicular secretion." In the 1930s it was done for rejuvenation, in the 1940s to prevent infection after prostate surgery.

The operation is performed under local. The patient needs only spare an hour from his day and spend longer than usual shaving that morning. Like all operations, it is more difficult than it looks. Each spermatic cord is exposed at the root of the penis, a slice of vas deferens cut, the ends sealed. Both sections go under the laboratory microscope. The surgeon may snip vein or tendonous muscle by mistake, disastrous when the patient revels in his new freedom (the record is two hours postoperatively, including lunch in Soho). Insisting the patient has a sperm-count before letting fly avoids the surgeon being sued for making his wife pregnant. The vasectomized virgin dons a tie invitingly lettered IOFB—I Only Fire Blanks. Intact males retaliate with IFLR, more puzzling and equally vulgar.

Vasectomy guillotines a man's reproductive life thirty years before its death from natural enfeeblement. The young husband resuming the nuptual couch, as incapable of fatherhood as a mysogynic eunuch, may later wish to change this piece of bed-room furniture. His joyful ability to plant without reaping may encourage it, in widening the circle of his feminine acquaint-ances. The stark new marriage demands the embellishment of children. He returns to his surgeon.

Restoring a vasectomy is more difficult than taping together plastic garden hose chewed by the dog. The fiddly operation of vaso-vasotomy may not work. It is unfortunate that we cannot install a stop-cock. Perhaps the solution is bottling some sperm pre-vasectomy, and laying it down in the freezer for enjoyment several years later, like home cooking.

My good friend and neighbor, distinguished doctor-writer David Delvin, wrote up his own vasectomy in the late seventies. As a moving example of self-sought tragedy it matches *Othello*.

The postoperative morning, disaster struck. The ligature slipped from his spermatic artery. What Australians call the family jewel-box began to swell. Within minutes, it resembled a coconut. Within hours, it matched a honeydew melon. By night-fall, it was indistinguishable from a soccer ball. By morning, the color deepened, and it could have passed for a London gentle-man's bowler hat.

The disabled doctor could reach the telephone across the room only on all fours, suspending the afflicted parts with a squash racket clutched beneath his breastbone. When young men at parties now cadge advice about a vasectomy, I simply clap them on the shoulder and bark, "Buy a squash racket!"

I do not envy Dr. Delvin's experience. Only his title. "Black-balled."

# 40

## DISASTROUS HABITS

### *Tom Brown's Schooldays*

Thomas Hughes' glorification of public school life appeared simultaneously in 1857 with Dr. William Acton's damnation of its popular-do-it-yourself activity.

> The frame is stunted and weak, the muscles underdeveloped, the eye is sunken and heavy, the complexion is sallow, pasty, or covered with spots of acne, the hands are damp and cold, and the skin moist. The boy shuns the society of others, creeps about alone, joins with repugnance in the amusements of his schoolfellows. He cannot look anyone in the face, and becomes careless in dress and uncleanly in person. His intellect has become sluggish and enfeebled, and if his evil habits are persisted in, he may end in becoming a drivelling idiot or a peevish valitudinarian. Such boys are to be seen in all stages of degeneration, but what we have described is but the result toward which they all are tending . . .

> The pale complexion, the emaciated form, the slouching gait, the clammy palm, the glassy or leaden eye, and the averted gaze, indicate the lunatic victim to this vice. Apathy, loss of memory, abeyancy of concentrative power and manifestation of mind generally, combined with loss of self-reliance, and indisposition for or impulsiveness of action, irritability of temper, and incoherence of

language, are the most characteristic mental phenomena of chronic dementia resulting from masturbation . . .

The man will and must pay the penalty for the errors of the boy; that for one that escapes, ten will suffer; that an awful risk attends abnormal substitutes for sexual intercourse; and that self-indulgence, long pursued, tends ultimately, if carried far enough, to early death or self-destruction.

Thus, "The Function and Disorders of the Reproductive Organs, in Childhood, Youth, Adult Age, and Advanced Life, Considered in their Physiological, Social and Moral Relations." Dr. Acton wrote as well, "Prostitution, Considered in its Moral, Social, and Sanitary Aspects, in London and other Large Cities and Garrison Towns, with Proposals for the Control and Prevention of its Attendant Evils." Also, "Unmarried Wet-Nurses."

I doubt if he would have appreciated Dorothy Parker's scriptural joke, when she named her untidy canary Onan.

# 41

## AND SO TO BED

### *Devilish Disaster*

On the rainy Monday afternoon of April 6, 1668, Samuel Pepys went to a cockfight, which he thought no great sport.

> And thence to the park in a hackney-coach, so would not go into the Tour, but round about the park and to the House, and there at the door eat and drank; whither came my Lady Kerneagy, of whom Creed tells me more perticulary: how her Lord, finding her and the Duke of York at the King's first coming in too kind, did get it out of her that he did dishonour him; and so he bid her continue to let him, and himself went to the foulest whore he could find, that he might get the pox; and did, and did give his wife it on purpose, that she (and he persuaded and threatened her that she should) might give it the Duke of York; which she did, and he did give it the Duchess; and since, all her children are thus sickly and infirm—which is the most pernicious and foul piece of revenge that ever I heard of. And he at this day owns it with great glory, and looks upon the Duke of York and the world with great content in the ampleness of his revenge.

This story told Pepys by the Earl of Sandwich's servant John Creed has been disclosed regularly since 1665, by the Comte de Gramont (who was Anthony Hamilton), by Gilbert Burnet (who was Bishop of Salisbury) and by a London doctor I met last week in a pub (who swore it happened in the 1960s to the wife of a Cabinet Minister).

# 42

## CLEANER LIVING

### *Nature Adores a Vacuum*

The loves of senior citizens and venerable monarchs usually provoke ridicule and pity, sometimes admiration and envy, always curiosity.

Every schoolboy sniggers over King David stricken in years, the fair young virgin Abishag lying in his bosom, "but the king knew her not"—which did not mean they were unacquainted.

King Solomon after his Queen of Sheba phase "loved many strange women."

A barefoot beggar maid affected King Cophetua so decisively that in robe and crown the king stept down and swore a royal oath: "This beggar maid shall be my queen!" Tennyson heard all about it.

King Charles II at 40 sired the Duke of St. Alban's with the help of pretty, witty Nell Gwynn, aged 20.

Many ageing men fall desperately in love with their vacuum cleaners. Particularly the Hoover "Dustette" model. These are mistresses more dangerous than Carmen in torrid Saville.

A London man was changing the plug of his "Dustette" in the nude while his wife was out shopping, when it inexplicably turned itself on. A railwayman was mysteriously caught in one that happened to be lying about buzzing in his signal box. Another man was hoovering a friend's stairs in a dressing gown, when the suction got him. Another in Denver, Colorado, was vacuuming his car in the back yard, dressed only in his underpants. The cleaner clogged, he sat on the back steps to free it, the motor started unexpectedly and drew him in, as a straw in the wind.

All ten recorded cases were between 55 and 75. All ended disastrously in hospital for suturing and skin grafting. The whirring fan of a "Dustette" seems a safe 6 inches inside, but the surgeon remarked, "They were driven to new lengths by the novelty of the experience."

Some gentlemen become affectionate toward the doorstep milk bottle, which unlike the real thing is liable to produce penis captivus. As an intern, I encountered a man impassioned of a stone hot-water bottle, the sort then warming beds in Britain's Dickensian country hotels. It was a stonemason's job rather than a surgeon's. As we guardedly chipped away the pottery, the patient commented only that it had seemed a good idea at the time.

Ladies have been enamored of briar pipes, cold-cream jars, the bust of Napoleon, bananas, three oranges (uninspired by Prokofiev). Men of experimental outlook have female vibrators torpedoing up their innards ("the oscillating umbilicus syndrome"). Treatment—let the battery run down.

The resourceful skill, the cheerful unreproach, which medicine applies to mankind's infinite idiosyncrasies is illustrated by the book which taught me surgery.

> The variety of foreign bodies which have found their way into the rectum is hardly less remarkable than the ingenuity displayed in their removal. A turnip has been delivered per anum by the use of obstetric forceps. A stick firmly impacted has been withdrawn by inserting a gimlet into its lower end. A tumbler, mouth looking downward, has several times been extracted by filling the interior with a wet plaster of Paris bandage, leaving the end of the bandage extruding, and allowing the plaster to set.

Do not mock the peccadillos of the old. Only with luck shall we live to enjoy them.

# 43

## BOOB BOOBS

### *A Thing of Beauty Is a Joy for Lawyers*

If you do not care for just the way you look tonight, a plastic surgeon can operate on you as efficiently as a fairy godmother on toads.

Take your choice of cut:

*Facelift.* Camouflage incision under hairline, pull taut, insert tuck, snip off selvedge. Eliminates the sags like wind in your sails.

*Nosebob.* All done from inside. Makes a classical feature of something fit only as a perch for glasses.

*Browbob.* Eliminates furrows by cut at nape of neck, scalp pulled back, surplus sliced, secured with metal staples as for sealing postal packets. Stops you looking worried.

*Boobbob.* Any shape from Rubens to Bernard Buffet, Picasso if you like.

*Wattlebob.* Turns old turkeys into fighting cocks.

*Bagbob.* Under eyes, cancels a lifetime's dissipation.

*Bumbob.* Goes with Tummy Tuck, Thigh Whittling, Fat Syphoning. Anything is preferable to dieting.

*Hair Transplant.* Replaces bald patches with flourishing ones, as returfing the lawn.

Plastic surgery like any other has its mistakes, but they are more obvious. The facelift droops with time, as an uneaten soufflê. Surgeons favor a standard, quick pert nose-job, and a woman is as infuriated encountering another wearing the same little nose as the same little dress. Boob-boosting is done with silicone implants, which can slop like sandbags and cause severe list to port or starboard. This once brought thunderous applause, occurring suddenly at the climax of a stripper's act.

Mrs. Virginia O'Hare of New York said she wanted a flat, sexy belly. The plastic surgeon left her navel 1½ inches off center. She sued him, won the disastrous damages of $650,000. This operative error is priced at $433,333 per inch, or over fifteen and a half million dollars a yard.

# 44

## Obstetrical Obsession
### *Maternal Mutilation*

A baby joyously enters the world much like a circus clown bursting head first through a paper hoop. The rips are immediately neatly stitched—gynecologists enjoy the Biblical appellation of sewers of tears in other men's fields.

To snip with scissors the stretched perineum, against which the baby is lustily butting, had seemed for years an elegant stroke of preventive medicine. No one amid the bustle and alarms of maternity thought twice about it, until the National Childbirth Trust in 1981 called this operation of episiotomy "A genital mutilation, the most common form of genital mutilation we have in the West."

The shocked comparison was to female circumcision, ceremonially performed in Central and East Africa on 10- to 14-year-old girls, one sweep of a sharp knife and white chicken feathers to dress the wound.

"Episiotomies are done much too casually and women are far too often teaching material for students," objected the NCT lady. Of 1,800 mothers studied, she discovered the two-thirds who suffered this unthinking obstetrical maneuver were twice as liable to severe pain the first week after delivery. More disastrously, many complained their sex lives were ruined for a year, causing marital disintegration.

This doomful diagnosis is contradicted by the oldest obstetrical story.

MIDWIFE: (*Visiting patient's home, surveying site of delivery five days afterward.*) Now, Mrs. Jones, I'm going to remove your episiotomy stitches—Mrs. Jones! They've gone!
PATIENT: Oh, my husband took them out.
MIDWIFE: (*Horrified.*) *Your husband took them out!*
PATIENT: Yes, Sister. He said they tickled.
   (*Collapse of stout nursing party.*)
Unfortunately, NCT seems to have no sense of humor.

# 45

# THE JOY (SLIGHTLY IMPAIRED)
## OF SEX

### *Boswell's Clap in 1763*

In the autumn of 1762, James Boswell was aged 22, priggish, puritanical, energetic, gregarious, vain, sceptical, witty, superstitious, hypochondriacal, suffering from an anxiety neurosis, and dreadfully randy.

He was black-haired, brown-eyed, muddy-complexioned, five foot six, and fat. He was the eldest son of a judge, Lord Auchinleck, who lived at Parliament Close near the Courthouse in Edinburgh, a city of granite morals, vaulted thought, freezing winds, and soggy cooking.

Lord Auchinleck was determined James should strut the family path through the law. He educated the youth with tutors, ordinands of the Church of Scotland, young men of impregnable gravity and impeccable bigotry. He sent him to the universities of both Edinburgh and Glasgow.

Lord Auchinleck regarded his son with an eighteenth-century father's natural suspicion. James Boswell attended the theater, danced attendance on actresses, published boyish verses in *The Scots Magazine*, frivolities to Lord Auchinleck equally despicable. Disinheriting the lad was infuriatingly frustrated by his own marriage contract (his wife Euphemia brought money into the family). He settled for a deed placing James under the control of trustees—chosen by himself—bribing him £100 a year to sign it.

A couple of years before, Boswell had run away to London, two and a half days on horseback, riding around the clock. He hankered to exchange the chilly stone-flagged corridors of Calvinism for the scented gaudy salons of the Roman Catholic Church, which received him at the Bavarian Chapel, Golden Square, Soho. He decided to enter a monastery in France. He met some remarkably jolly fellows and delightfully easygoing girls, and decided against it. After three months, his father demanded he come home.

Lord Auchinleck had one sure, tried way of submitting wayward James to vocational discipline and domestic immobility for life. He would get him married. Boswell took tea with earnestly eligible young ladies in the drawing room, his pleasure with servant girls in the attic. (He fathered Peggy Doig's child, but gave her £10 to cover costs.) He informed Lord Auchinleck he desired a commission in His Majesty's Footguards. This was not to restore filial probity, but an unchallengeable reason for living permanently in London.

He quit Edinburg society—as narrow as its Wynds, as dull as its weather, as severe as its sermons, as prying as its excisemen's lanterns—at ten in the morning of Monday, November 15, 1762. His chaise rattled down the High Street, the chairmen sagging beneath heavy Sedans seeming to exclaim, "God prosper long our noble Boswell!" The journey took four days and cost £11.

Boswell stayed in Pall Mall with his friend Andrew Douglas, a Scottish naval surgeon—apprentice-trained, not a bookish member of Henry VIII's Royal College. Boswell dropped joyously into the gossipy, chaffing, tippling, informed, prejudiced, contentious, allusive, humorous male society crowding the scorching fires of London chop-houses and coffee-houses. But what was an evening's scintillating conversation compared to five delightful minutes with a girl?

Girls were as available as the chops and claret, at the same prices. They paraded the jostling, dung-spattered, lampless Strand north of the Thames, swarmed the Haymarket alongside the Royal Opera House, filled St. James's Park under its orderly trees drilled from the Horse Guards to Buckingham House. Boswell took one up an alley off the Strand "with the intention to enjoy her in armor." She was at work ill-equipped. "She wondered at my size, and said if I ever took a girl's maidenhead, I would make her squeak. I gave her a shilling, and had enough command of myself to let her go without touching her. I afterward trembled at the danger I had escaped. I resolved to wait cheerfully till I got some safe girl or was liked by some woman of fashion."

The armor was either of linen or a sheep's caecum, the blind end of intestine that extrudes the appendix. The sheep's gut was soaked in alkaline lye, everted, scraped, pickled in burning brimstone, washed with soap, blown up, trimmed to eight inches and threaded at the base with a pretty ribbon for show (officers could order their regimental colors).

The best quality—"Baudruches fines"—were fashioned on oiled molds, scented with essences, polished with glass rods. The "Superfine Double" was two caecums gummed together. You bought them from Mrs. Phillips at the sign of the Golden Fan and Rising Sun at Orange Court in Leicester Fields, off Piccadilly. Casanova called them English overcoats, and blew them up to send his ladies into fits.

For one sex, they avoided "the big belly and the squawling brat." For the other,

Happy the Man, who in his Pocket keeps,
Whether with Green or Scarlet Ribband bound,
A well-made Condom He, nor dreads the Ills
Of Shankers or Cordee, or Buboes Dire!

Mrs. Douglas talked too much. Boswell moved to Downing Street, forty guineas a year for an upstairs room and use of the parlor all forenoon. The organ that won knowledgeable acclaim remained the tail which wagged the dog. Even in church he laid plans for having women "from the splendid Madam at fifty guineas a night, down to the civil nymph with white-thread stockings who tramps the Strand," though without disturbing his piety.

In St. James's park with pretty, seventeen-year-old Elizabeth Parker, "for the first time did I engage in armor, which I found but a dull satisfaction." (A Yorkshireman once compared it to washing your feet with your boots on.) His open-air harem yielded also an ugly, skinny, sullen girl who stank of gin, and strong, plump, good-humored Nanny Baker. In our present Prime Minister's garden he enjoyed fresh, agreeable Alice Gibbs—unarmored, she urged it was so much nicer without and she was as clean as the Queen of England. Fool, fool! he told himself next morning. To have believed one of those abandoned, deceitful wretches! He anticipated the rebuke from Brigadier Mitchner of the Royal Army Medical Corps to World War II troops: "Some of you fellows put your private parts where I wouldn't stick the ferrule of my umbrella."

Boswell relished what is technically known as a knee-trembler with a jolly young damsel on Westminster Bridge. He met in the Strand "a monstrous big whore," took her to a nearby inn where "she displayed to me all the parts of her enormous carcas," but found her avarice as large as her arse and "walked off with the gravity of a Barcelonian bishop." He tried making amends with a little girl up an alley, but could not rise to it.

He almost got a free one from Miss Watts, the *grande horizontale* of the Shakespeare tavern, but a paying customer took priority. He collected instead a couple of pretty little girls in Covent Garden and had them over a bottle of sherry, in order of seniority. On King George III's birthday he dressed in old clothes to spy the night's celebrations, picked up a surly girl in the Park, called himself a barber, and settled for sixpence, dangled his linen armor in the Park canal for comfort, had an inconclusive knee-trembler with a wench in the Strand (six pence), tried getting it free in Whitehall, and reached home at two, much fatigued.

A girl in Whitehall picked his pocket. He had one in the Temple, haunt of lawyers, in the afternoon. A fine fresh lass tapped his shoulder in the Strand, an officer's daughter, born in Gibraltar, irresistible. Then he gloomily left the familiar frolics of London to tour the Continent. Perhaps he consoled himself, Tomorrow to fresh whores and pussies new.

Each jig to the carefree music of nightingales brought the vultures of remorse roosting on his morning bedposts. He was revolted at low street debauchery, shocked at intimate union with sluts, determined to do it no more—for 25 days at the longest, two at the least. The frankness of Boswell's frailty is charming. We do not care to admit our own even with regard to bleaker activities like avoiding potatoes.

He longed for a healthy well-bred girl. Amid his boisterous whoring he found one. Her name was Mrs. Lewis.

Louisa was an actress. She had played the Queen in *Hamlet*. She was 24, pretty, tall, deep-bosomed, good-natured, vivacious, with "an enchanting languish in her eyes." Her husband was Charles Standen, a strolling player who had strolled off. Boswell called for tea. They talked of love, philosophically. He stayed till eight. She hoped he would come again.

He was back next morning. He had woken in a frenzy of love. He declared it bashfully, saying he sought only agreeable conversation and tea. She said he was always welcome. He proclaimed never to contemplate copulation with a woman he did not love. She agreed, adding she was no Platonist. To a man of Boswell's fire, that was a proposition. He kissed her hand and asked how about it. She said, give me time. He mentioned that he was obliged to live with great economy.

He was back after breakfast. She borrowed two guineas off him.

Boswell reckoned the loan a bargain. It would cost more, being cured of something caught from a whore. How about tomorrow? he suggested. She was sick-visiting. Well, the day after? Perhaps. She sang for him.

He arrived two mornings later, exclaimed how neat her lodgings were and threw open the bedroom door to look. She made him sit down and talk of religion. He jumped up, crying, "You are above the finesse of your sex!" (Be sure always to make a woman better than her sex, he noted that night in his diary.) She asked for more time. *When?* he exclaimed frantically. Friday.

He went home to bread and cheese. It was all he could afford after lending her the two guineas.

On Friday she had second thoughts. He distractedly probed her objections, all as unassailably unsatisfying as any housewife's bedtime headache. He promised in desperation to support any windfall fruit of their union. She told him to cool off for a week.

The week went. He pulled up her petticoats. "Good heaven, sir!" "Madam, I cannot help it, I adore you!" She pressed him to her bosom. "Oh, Mr. Boswell!" They fixed on Sunday afternoon, when her landlady was at church.

Wisely not wishing to miss Sunday dinner (roast beef and hot apple pie), Boswell ate an hour early and hurried to Louisa at three. He got the penile equivalent of cold feet. Supposing he was impotent? His anxiety neurosis worsened the probability. She tactfully pretended to forget the agenda of their meeting. He resolutely clutched her alabaster breasts and kissed her delicious lips and led her fluttering into the bedroom. Then her bloody landlady came in. *And* her brother. Boswell cleared out and went to church.

On Monday, Louisa wanted even more time. Tuesday, she fixed Saturday night. She would have Sunday to get over it. Boswell reserved a room at the Black Lion in Water Lane off the Old Bailey, as Mr. and Mrs. Digges. On Friday, she told him she had started her period.

Ten days of coquettish and physiological frustration ended at eight o'clock on Wednesday night, when Louisa met him in the Piazzas of Covent Garden. A hackney coach waited, with drawn blinds. They arrived at the Black Lion beside Apothecaries Hall, faking the end of a long journey, even to macaroons for munching *en route*.

The couple supped. They drank a few glasses. The maid put on the sheets, well aired. They ordered mulled port floating with fruit for afterward. Boswell climbed into bed like the challenger climbing into the ring with the champ. He was clasped in her snowy arms and pressed to her milk-white bosom. She was the exquisite mixture of delicacy and wantonness. He did it five times. She said that was three over par. He dozed, fantasizing doing it with other women of his acquaintance. They rose at ten and ate a hearty breakfast. They left by hackney coach and parted in Soho Square.

Five days passed. He felt "a little heat in the members of my body sacred to Cupid." Idle fears! He called on Louisa and did it again. Next evening he was out with the boys, to dinner, the play, supper, enormous fun. He got home. "Too, too plain was Signor Gonorrhoea."

He was appalled. A dose from a tart was losing a bet in a lively game. From a lady like Louisa, it was like finding yourself mugged in the confessional. "Those damned twinges, that scald-ing heat, and that deep-tinged loathsome matter . . ." His dis-charge was as the blood on Brutus's dagger to dying Caesar. He went to breakfast with Andrew Douglas.

Boswell was familiar with the symptoms. He caught his first dose on the earlier jaunt to London, next year he "catch'd a Tartar" in Edinburgh. Douglas prescribed confinement to his room, rest, a skimpy diet, aperients, and bloodletting. He had hoped for free treatment, but Douglas charged five guineas. Bos-well discovered perplexedly, "The same man as a friend and a surgeon exhibits two very opposite characters." It was irksome, inhibiting, infuriating. Particularly in scotching his plan shortly to have a go at a Lady Mirabel.

Boswell called on Louisa. He was dignified, bitter, incisive, sorrowful, noble. So would the head of John the Baptist have addressed Salome. She grew pale and atremble. She passionately denied ever having the clap—well, not for fifteen months. He left with icy finality. She falteringly asked if she might continue asking after his health. "'Madam,' said I, archly, 'I fancy it will be needless for some weeks.'" He decided she was a most consum-mate dissembling whore.

Like the syphilitic spirochaete of the Emperor Frederick III, Louisa's gonococcus only slept, to awaken at a lover's caress.

Boswell gave out that he had gone to the country. He suffered bouts of fever so wretched that he glimpsed death. He anguished that his testicle might swell again. He dreamed of Douglas at his bedside pronouncing, "This is a damned difficult case." After five weeks, the illness was reduced to a scanty discharge and Douglas freed him. It was a textbook case of untreated gonorrhoea.

An excoriating letter to Louisa demanded his two guineas back. "If you are not rendered callous by a long course of disguised wickedness, I should think the consideration of your deceit and baseness, your corruption both of body and mind, would be a very severe punishment." Her servant girl brought a package, unad-dressed, without a written word. Boswell relented. Had he been too harsh? He contemplated sending the money back. He decided against it. After all, "I had come off two guineas better than I expected."

On May 16, 1763, Boswell met Samuel Johnson. This relationship would have kept many another man's mind off women for life. Not Boswell. He had 16 more attacks of clap, five illegitimate children, and got the crabs in Venice. "One night of Irish extravagance" in Dublin had him on Kennedy's Lisbon Diet Drink (sasparilla, sassafras, liquorice, guaiac wood, half a guinea a pint). His urinary passages needed irrigation with vitriol, nitrous acid, mercury salts, and lead. Ouch. On January 31, 1770, he wrote, "Earle's: sounded: almost fainted." The inevitable stricture had developed, to be periodically dilated with metal rods passed up his penis.

On May 14, 1795, Boswell collapsed at a dinner of the Literary Club and was carried home. He could not pass urine. An abscess had developed in his prostate. He died of kidney failure at 2 A.M. on May 19. At 29 he had married his cousin, who had seven children and three miscarriages.

Boswell's contemporary and counterpart Nicolas Chamfort wrote, *l'amour, tel qu'il existe dans la société, n'est que l'échange de deux fantasies et le contact de deux épidermes*. Love, as it exists in society, is only the exchange of two fantasies and the contact of two epidermises.

It was the only frailty Boswell never confessed. He was too romantic to recognize it.

# 46

## THE JOY (NAVAL FASHION) OF SEX
### *Disastrous Effect of Shore Leave*

United States Navy routine, 1913:

> In those who have been exposed to infection the entire penis is scrubbed with liquid soap and water for several minutes, and then washed with mercuric perchloride lotion 1:2000. Abrasions are sprayed with hydrogen peroxide. Two urethral injections of argyrol (10%) are then given and retained for five minutes. The whole penis is then rubbed with 33% calomel ointment which is kept on for several hours.

*—The Medical Annual.*

# Part Ten

# FINAL DIAGNOSIS

# 47

# 101 USES OF A DEAD POPE

## *Disaster on Judgment Day*

After the appalling attack outside St. Peter's on May 13, 1981, Pope John Paul II was rushed to the Gemelli Clinic, where Dr. Giancarlo Castiglioni, in a 4 hour 10 minute operation, removed two bullets and the damaged sections of intestine.

The disposal of these scraps was more delicately circumspect than bits of ourselves, or of President Reagan in the George Washington University Hospital six weeks earlier.

Tissue excised in the operating theater is ordinarily dropped into a stainless steel dish held by the scrub nurse, tipped into a plastic sack, and incinerated with the day's debris. One Harley Street throat surgeon pocketed the tonsils and adenoids, swearing they worked wonders on his strawberry beds. But the Vicar of Christ must be reverenced, even in fragments.

His Holiness's pieces of gut were taken to the baroque church of Santi Vincenzo ed Anastasio, opposite the Trevi fountain. This was rebuilt in 1630, parish church of the next door Palazzo del Quirinale. The crypt contains the sacra praecordia. Here repose the entrails removed during embalming of all popes from Sixtus V (died August 27, 1590). They are kept in large terracotta jars. The general public is not admitted.

The praecordium is an everyday clinical term for the area of chest over the heart. The Latin is anatomically imprecise, meaning bowels, stomach, diaphragm. Ecclesiastically it conveys "the holy region before the heart" or "the sacred internal organs." The words carry a mystical meaning beyond the workmanlike minds of those who every day commit "no small presumption to dismember the image of God"—as Queen Elizabeth I's surgeon, John Woodall, put it. Medically, a dead pope is no different from a dead poacher.

The traumatized organs of our present vigorous pope must wait many years to be joined by their healthy fellows. Three dozen popes have been embalmed since Sixtus V, their entrails deposited in the Piazza di Trevi, their husks borne to the Vatican Grottoes under St. Peter's. When jolly Pope John Paul I, who died after 33 days, was kept too long above ground in a hot Roman September—so that his funeral might be captured live for U.S. prime time TV—the deficiences of a botched embalming job grew noisomely noticeable.

Come Judgment Day, trunk and organs will be united, that a shining procession of popes may parade past the seat of the Almighty. This is the well-publicized divine plan for us all. But God made man in his image, which suggests a celestial snafu when the Last Trump blows. Judgment Day will be dreadfully confusing, with the jostling and the trumpets and the wails of the sinners, as Michaelangelo indicated with customary vision on the east wall of the Sistine Chapel. The angelic reassembly of the Holy Fathers will be a more distracted operation than the slick mechanisms of Detroit.

"Michael," comes the heavenly intercom a mile and a half across Rome from the Piazza di Trevi to the Piazza San Pietro. "Can you help me, old man? I seem to have got the right kidney of Clement IX left over down here."

"Gee, I'm sorry, Philip. But I guess I'm fully equipped kidney-wise over here."

"But Mike, how *is* Clement IX? I mean, does he look like a pope with only one kidney?"

"Clement looks fine, Phil, absolutely dinky. He's enjoying his breakfast. Nothing like lying around since 1669 to give a man an appetite."

"Mike, old chap. Are you sure he *is* Clement IX?"

"Recognize him anywhere, Phil."

"I mean, you haven't got the wrong head on him?"

"Hey! Wait a minute. So I have! It's eating Benedict XIII's eggs benedict. Fancy that, eh? I'll just move 'em around . . . excuse me, Your Holiness. Thanks a lot. Say, Phil?"

"Yes, Mike?"

"Got Innocent XI's left leg out there by any chance? You could fly it in."

"Sorry, Mike. Best I can do is Alexander VII's pancreas. Are you sure, old chap, that Innocent XI had a left leg?"

"Maybe there *was* a one-legged pope, Phil, but I've sure never heard of one with three arms, like Leo XI at this moment."

"Look, be an angel and let me have Urban VIII back. Inside, he's Gregory XIV."

I expect it will be all right on the Day.

# 48

## THE FINAL WORD

### *Still Dodgy*

Why don't you say it? Of course he's dead. But you must be sure. Once said it can't be unsaid.... It leaves you with an uneasy feeling that after half an hour in the Chapel of Rest the patient will sit up and ask for a large Scotch without ice.

—A Welsh GP

At noon on November 21, 1741, Jane Brown, delirious with smallpox, threw herself into the New River at Islington in north London. She was noticed floating face down by an old man on the opposite bank, who tottered off to raise the alarm at the Crown alehouse, some way off.

The only problem for the citizens who dragged her out was the right parish to bury her—Islington or next door Clerkenwell. After a wrangle, they had Bill Stevens the gravedigger and Tom Bull the parish pallbearer carry the corpse to Clerkenwell's St. James's workhouse. It was frosty. Bill slipped on the grass. The body fell. Raising it up again, they heard a groan.

The workhouse master was unimpressed. He laid Jane on the lid of the parish coffin in the cold outside the infirmary door, ordained spot for inmates awaiting burial. A human body is always an object of interest. A passer-by noticed her upper lip quiver. They put her to bed and sent for Mr. Oborne, surgeon and apothecary.

It was then three in the afternoon. He found her cold, pulseless, distended. He effected urgent resuscitation with spirit of hartshorn in warm water. They rubbed her with coarse cloths. She croaked. She belched. Up came the river water. They tipped her head-down, it ran everywhere.

Mr. Oborne next administered sliced ginger in mountain wine, but she seemed to have died again. He sent urgently for a hot flannel petticoat. Jane's jaw trembled, she rumbled, belched mightily, moved an arm. More ginger and wine. Her pulse fluttered. They wrapped her all over in warm flannel, the emergency medicines arrived, they gave her Raleigh's confection and tincture of cardamom. At eight, she was supping off broth and bread.

Next morning Jane felt splendid, if sore all over. In a week she was walking around the ward, complaining only of everlasting hunger. Her smallpox got better, too.

In 1773, Patrick Redmond, condemned for robbery, was hanged on an Irish gallows for 29 minutes by the stopwatch. He was cut down, hastened by friends to nearby fields as the sheriff retired, given a tobacco clyster and stimulated with lighted pipes. The mob rubbed his limbs in relays from two in the afternoon until six, when his neck encouragingly began to bleed. The sheriff heard of the insolent wake, the mob whisked their patient from under his nose, kept him two days on warm brandy and water lying on stable hay, sped him off to avoid capture. Patrick was later said to be fine in County Clare.

A Swedish gardener in 1676, upright for 16 hours in 60 feet of freezing water at Tronningholm, was restored to life by heat from the stove. The Russians were always suffocating themselves from stoves, but revived when rolled in the snow. When Ann Green was hanged at Oxford in 1650, her corpse was handled so roughly it woke her up. Doctors think she had an ossified larynx.

The bell gloomily tolls for all mankind, the messenger galloping up, as the firing squad cocks its rifles, cheerfully reprieves us all.

But even Lazarus died sometime.

# 49

## GREATEST DISASTER OF ALL

### *Pressing Proclivity to Procreate*

The world population increases by one million every Monday to Friday.

It took from cavemen to 1830 to reach 1,000 million, from the crinoline to the Charleston to reach 2,000 million, from Hitler to Krushchev to reach 3,000 million, from the Beatles to Mrs. Thatcher to reach 4,000 million.

By 2112 it will level out at 10,500 million, two and a half times what it is now. Or perhaps at 14,200 million in 2132, the United Nations is not sure. Though with luck, we might be only 8,000 million in 2040. The roads will still be dreadfully busy.

The increase will be lopsided. In 2110, the rich countries will be only 13 percent of the global population, against 24 percent today. Europe will stop increasing itself in 2030, and America in 2060. The Third World will then have tripled itself, to 9,100 million.

"While imbalances created by poverty, malnutrition, or ill-health persist," say the United Nations," the social tensions arising out of population pressures will permeate every aspect of life on earth."

Luckily, we are steadily killing ourselves and hardly noticing it.

"As much as 50 percent of mortality from the 10 leading causes of death in the United States can be traced to lifestyle," says the

U.S. National Institute of Medicine. Three-quarters of Americans die from heart and circulatory disease, cancer, accidents, or violence, which they bring upon themselves with cigarettes (one-third of Americans over 19 smoke), alcohol (134 million drink, often too much), drugs, driving, quack medicines, and "maladaptive responses to social pressures."

The rich nations *must* respond to idealistic urgings and help the poor ones. Once the benefits of civilization come to Africa and Southern Asia, they will kill themselves off just as eagerly.

# 50

## DISASTROUS END

Man's activities have been hopelessly open to disaster since that calamitous business of the serpent in the Garden of Eden. Best treatment is to admit, to analyze, to avoid. Medicine readily confesses its share. But what a disaster, were there no doctors amid the world's unending catalogue of disasters.

> The profession of medicine and surgery must always rank as the most noble that man can adopt. The spectacle of a doctor in action among soldiers (or sailors) in equal danger with equal courage, saving life where all others are taking it, allaying pain where all others are causing it, is one which must always seem glorious, whether to God or man.

The writer brought us through the greatest disaster of this century.

Thank you, Sir Winston.

If you can meet with Triumph and Disaster
And treat those two imposters just the same . . .
                                        —*Rudyard Kipling*

# REFERENCES

1. Triple Knock-Out
   Cock, W. F., "The First Operation under Ether in Europe,"
   *University College Hospital Magazine* 1 (1911): 127-44.
   Flemming, P., "Robert Liston, the First Professor of Clinical
   Surgery at UCH," *University College Hospital Magazine* 1
   (1926): 176–85.
2. The Emperor's Sore Throat
   *Financial Times,* January 23, 1982.
   Holland, C., *The Notebooks of a Spinster Lady, 1878–1903,*
   London: Cassel, 1919, p. 268.
   Stevenson, R. S., *Morell Mackenzie,* London: Heinemann,
   1946.
3. Kinky Kinks
   Layton, T. B., *Sir William Arbuthnot Lane, Bt,* Edinburgh:
   Livingstone, 1956.
   Shaw, George Bernard, *The Doctor's Dilemma,* 1906, New
   York: Garland, 1981.
4. The Tender Trap
   *Chatelaine,* April 1976.
5. Surgical Souvenirs
   *The Medical Defence Union Annual Report,* 1980, p. 20.
6. The King Is Dead
   *British Medical Journal* i (1910): 1557–60.
   Guthrie, D., *A History of Medicine,* 2nd ed., London: Nelson,
   1958.

Latham, R., and Matthews, W., eds., *The Diary of Samuel Pepys,* Vol. 4, Berkeley: University of California Press, 1972.

Miller, J., *The Body in Question,* New York: Random House, 1979.

7. The Decline and Fall of Edward Gibbon

Dale, P. M., *Medical Biographies,* Norman: University of Oklahoma Press, 1952, pp. 112–17.

Gibbon, Edward, *Autobiography,* Oxford: University Press, 1907.

8. The Sack-'Em-Up Men

Guthrie, D., *A History of Medicine,* 2nd ed., London: Nelson, 1958.

Roughhead, W., *Burke and Hare (trial),* Edinburgh: Hodge, 1921.

Walbrook, H. M., *Murders and Murder Trials 1812–1912,* London: Constable, 1932.

9. *Rien Ne Va Plus*

Griffith, E. F., *Doctors by Themselves,* London: Cassell, 1951, p. 68.

11. Clubland Doctor

Griffith, E. F., *Doctors by Themselves,* London: Cassell, 1951, p. 63.

12. Disastrous Motherhood

Holmes, O. W., "On the Contagiousness of Puerperal Fever," *New England Quarterly Journal of Medicine, Boston* i (1842–43): 503–30.

13. Design for Living

*Sunday Times, The,* (London) January 31, 1982.

*Times, The,* (London) January 23, March 18, 1982.

Woodham-Smith, C., *Florence Nightingale,* Harmondsworth: Penguin, 1955.

14. Catastrophe

*Observer,* April 25, 1982.

15. Rude Awakening

*The Medical Defence Union Annual Report,* 1980, p. 55.

16. Typhoid Mary

Kellock, I. A., "The Curious Career of 'Typhoid Mary,'"

*Manchester University Medical School Gazette* 34 (1955): 133–36.

"Strange Fever," *MD*, 13 (1969): 220–26.

17. St. Anthony's Fire

*British Medical Journal*, ii (1951): 596.

Brown, P. W. F., "Bread Poisoning," *Notes & Queries* 4 (1957): 6–7.

Caporael, L. R., "Ergotism: The Satan Loosed in Salem?" *Science* 192 (1976): 21–26.

Gabbai, Lisbonne, and Pourquier, "Ergot Poisoning at Pont St. Esprit," *British Medical Journal* ii (1951): 650–51.

Spanos, N. P., and Gottlieb, J., "Ergotism and the Salem Village Witch Trials," *Science* 194 (1976): 1390–94.

Van Zwanenberg, D., "A 'Singular calamity,'" *Medical History* 17 (1973): 204–7.

18. Luckless Lübeck

Dubois, R., and Dubois, J., *The White Plague*, London: Gollancz, 1953.

Irvine, K. N., *BCG Vaccination in Theory and Practice*, Oxford: Blackwell, 1949.

Trollope, Anthony, *An Autobiography*, Edinburgh and London: Blackwood, 1883.

19. Bitter Victory

Beveridge, W. I. B., *Influenza: The Last Great Plague*, New York: Neale Watson Academic Pubns, 1977, pp. 30–33, 40–44.

Hoehling, A. A., *The Great Epidemic*, Boston: Little, Brown, 1961, p. 77.

Katz, R. S., "Flu, 1918–19: A Further Study in Mortality," *Bulletin of the History of Medicine* 51 (1977): 617–19.

Osborn, J. E., *History, Science and Politics: Influenza in America, 1918-1976*, New York: Prodist, 1977, pp. 4–13.

20. The Green Monkeys

*Trials of War Criminals Before the Nuremberg Military Tribunals Under Control Council Law No. 10*, Vol. 7, Washington: 1952. Trial of Professor Hörlein, p. 245.

Vella, E. E., "Marburg Virus Disease," *Update*, January 1977.

21. The Black Death

Ziegler, P., *The Black Death,* New York: Harper and Row, 1971.
23. Transatlantic Disaster
     Garrison, F. H., *History of Medicine,* 4th ed., Philadelphia: Saunders, 1929, pp. 189–92.
     Guthrie, D., *A History of Medicine,* 2nd ed., London: Nelson, 1958, pp. 164–65.
24. Calamity in the Cupboard
     Hornadge, B., ed., *The Ugly Australian,* Sydney: Bacchus Books, 1976, pp. 118, 124.
     Murphy, K. J., "Bilateral Renal Calculi and Aminoaciduria after Excessive Intake of Worcestershire Sauce," *Lancet* ii (1967): 401-2.
     *Times, The,* (London) August 18, 1967.
25. One in the Eye
     Archer, D., and Galloway, N., "Champagne-cork Injury to the Eye," *Lancet* ii (1967): 487–89.
26. Scurvy Treatment
     Cyriax, R. J., *Sir John Franklin's Last Arctic Expedition,* London: Methuen, 1939.
     Drummond, J. C., and Wilbraham, A., *The Englishman's Food,* 2nd ed., London: Cape, 1957.
     Orwell, G., *The Road to Wigan Pier,* London: Gollancz, 1937.
27. Sandwich Disaster
     *British Medical Journal* ii (1922): 394, 481, 527–28.
     *Times, The.* (London) August 18, 19, 21, 23, 25, 26, 1922; September 5, 6, 7, 8, 1922.
28. Doctor Death
     Browne, D. G., and Tullett, E. V., *Bernard Spilsbury,* London: Harrap, 1951.
     *Dictionary of National Biography, 1941-1950.*
     Orwell, G., "Decline of the English Murder," *Collected Essays, Journalism and Letters,* Vol. 4, Harmondsworth: Penguin, 1970, pp. 124–28.
     *Punch* 174 (1928): 305.
29. Ironing Out the Bugs in Panama
     Scott, H. H., *A History of Tropical Medicine,* London: Arnold, 1939.

30. Untreasured Island
   *Sunday Times, The,* (London) April 19, 1981.
   *Times, The,* (London) May 25, 1981.
31. Suffer the Little Children
   Baker, I. A. et al., "School Milk and Growth in Primary Schoolchildren," *Lancet* ii (1978): 575.
   *Sunday Times, The,* (London) September 10, 1978.
   *Times, The,* (London) September 2, October 1, 1981.
32. Disastrous Disasters
   Sloan, S., "Just Another Disaster," *World Medicine,* January 11, 1978.
   *Sunday Times, The,* (London), June 25, 1978.
33. The Dying Art
   Duff, C., *A Handbook on Hanging,* London: Cayme Press, 1928.
   Healey, T., "The Good Dr. Guillotin and His Humane Machine," *World Medicine,* April 5, 1978, pp. 61-71.
   Maugham, W. S., *A Writer's Notebook,* London: Heinemann, 1949, p. 254.
   Smith, S., *Forensic Medicine,* 8th ed., London: Churchill, 1945, p. 258.
   Soubiran, A., *The Good Doctor Guillotin,* London: Souvenir Press, 1964, p. 167.
   Weiner, D. B., "The Real Doctor Guillotin," *Journal of the American Medical Association,* April 3, 1972, pp. 85-89.
34. A Touch of Class
   Garrison, F. H., *History of Medicine,* 4th ed., Philadelphia: Saunders, 1929.
35. Beachy Head
   Irvine, M., "What Causes Death?" *World Medicine,* January 9, 1982.
   Surtees, S. J., "Suicide and Accidental Death at Beachy Head," *British Medical Journal* i (1982): 321-24.
   *Times, The,* (London) May 29, 1982.
36. It's a Cruel World
   *Asbestos: Financial Times,* June 22, 1982.
   *Dogs: The Times* (London), May 22, 1981. May 26, 1982.
   *Fungi: The Times* (London), September 16, 17, 1981.

*Glue: The Times* (London), September 4, 1981.

*Iatrogenesis: The Times* (London), April 16, 1981.

*Jail:* Garrison, F. H., *History of Medicine,* 4th ed., Philadelphia: Saunders, 1921, pp. 242–43.

*Melancholy: The Times* (London), May 12, 1982.

*Nature: Daily Telegraph,* September 20, 1979.

*Oranges:* Bowsher, W. G., and Kenyon, G. S., "Accidental Oropharyngeal Injury," *British Medical Journal* i (1982): 1752.

*Pot: The Times* (London), June 10, 1982.

*Risks: Financial Times,* September 5, 1981.

*Sheep: The Times* (London), July 2, 1981.

*Urea: Financial Times,* June 10, 1982.

*Video:* Daneshmend, T. K., and Campbell, M. J., "Dark Warrior Epilepsy," *British Medical Journal* i (1982): 1751–52.

*Xmas: Observer,* May 23, 1982.

37. Love Locked In

    Taylor, F. K., *British Medical Journal* ii (1979): 977–78.

38. Breaking It Off

    Johnson, G. R., and Corriere, J. N., "Partial Priapism," *Journal of Urology* 124 (1980): 147.

39. The Most Unkindest Cut of All

    Delvin, D., "Blackballed," *World Medicine,* June 28, 1978, p. 134.

    Vessey, M., Lawless, M., and Yeates, D., "Efficacy of Different Contraceptive Methods," *Lancet* i (1982): 841–42.

    Walsham, W. J., and Spencer, W. G., *Surgery: Its Theory and Practice,* 8th ed., London: Churchill, 1903, p. 1005.

41. And So to Bed

    Latham, R., and Matthews, W., eds., *The Diary of Samuel Pepys,* Vol. 9, Berkeley: University of California Press, 1976.

42. Cleaner Living

    Bailey, H., and Love, R. J. M., *A Short Practice of Surgery,* 6th ed., London: Lewis, 1943, p. 399.

    Citron, N. D., and Wade, P. J., "Penile Injuries from Vacuum Cleaners," *British Medical Journal* ii (1980): 26.

    Fox, M., and Barrett, E. L., "'Vacuum Cleaner Injury' of the Penis," *British Medical Journal* ii (1960): 1942.

Zufall, R., "Laceration of the Penis from Hand Vacuum Cleaners," *Journal of the American Medical Association* 224 (1973): 630.

43. Boob Boobs
*Daily Telegraph,* June 6, 1979.

44. Obstetrical Obsession
*Times, The* (London), September 25, 1981.

45. The Joy (Slightly Impaired) of Sex
Freyer, P., *The Birth Controllers,* London: Secker and Warburg, 1965.

Ober, W. B., *Boswell's Clap and Other Essays,* Carbondale and Edwardsville: Southern Illinois University Press, 1979.

Pottle, A. F., ed., *Boswell's London Journal, 1762-1763,* London: Heinemann, 1950.

46. The Joy (Naval Fashion) of Sex
*World Medicine,* May 30, 1981, p. 58.

47. 101 Uses of a Dead Pope
*Daily Telegraph,* May 14, 1981.

48. The Final Word
Humphreys, R., "Diagnosing Death," *World Medicine,* June 14, 1980, p. 55.

Payne, J. P., "On the Resuscitation of the Apparently Dead," *Annals of the Royal College of Surgeons of England* 45 (1964): 98.

Schuster, N. H., "The Emperor of Russia and the Royal Humane Society," *Journal of the Royal College of Practitioners* 21 (1971): 634.

Wood, S., "Resuscitation in 1741," *British Medical Journal* ii (1951): 671.

49. Greatest Disaster of All
*Times, The* (London), June 17, 1981, July 10, 1982.

50. Disastrous End
Roddis, L. H., *James Lind,* New York: Schuman, 1950, p. 3.